Marijuana Impaired Youths

A Clinical Handbook for Counselors, Mentors, Teachers and Parents.

By

Dr. Kay Wachuku

ISBN: 1-4140-6562-0 (e-book)
ISBN: 1-4140-6561-2 (Paperback)

Library of Congress Control Number: 2004090537

This book is printed on acid free paper.

Printed in the United States of America
Bloomington, IN

1stBooks – rev. 02/07/04

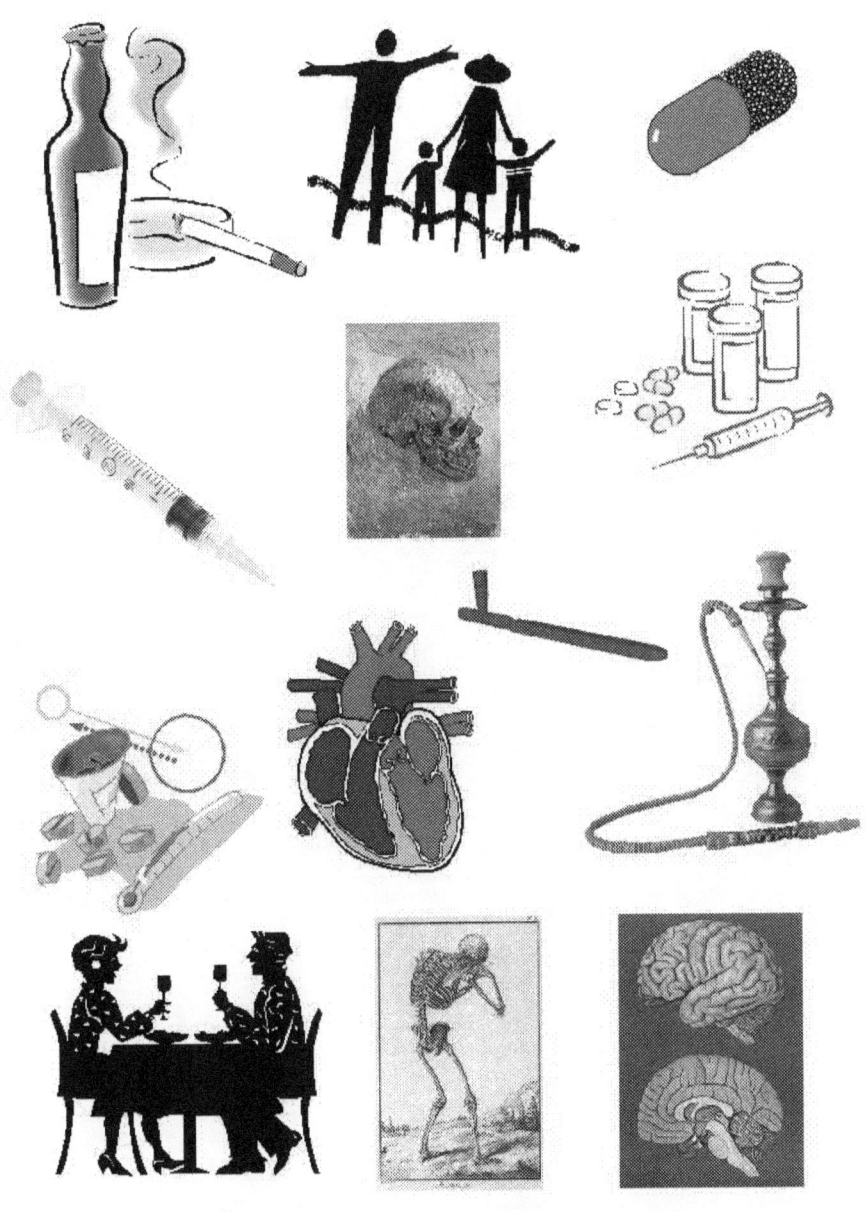

Dedicated to Sonnia (Nia) Wachuku

TABLE OF CONTENTS

Preface vii
Acknowledgements.. xi

1. Introduction: This Addiction Thing................................. 1
2. Addiction: Disease Or Social Maladjustment?....................... 8
   What Is Addiction? 10
   Genetic Predisposition To Addiction............................... 14
   Racial Predisposition To Alcoholism 17
   Genetic Predesposition To Other Drugs 18
   Socio-Psychology Of Youth Marijuana Addiction............... 26
   Socio-Cultural Addiction.. 31
3. Denial: Stumbling Block In Youth Addiction Treatment...... 36
   Self-Defeating Behavior (Sdb) Syndrome 38
   Terminal Uniqueness Syndrome.................................... 42
   Ed's Story 47
4. Building Therapeutic Alliance..................................... 51
   Youths In Treatment Demand 'Respekt' 53
   Leon's Story... 53
   Nicole's Story 55
   Mario's Story 57
   Youths In Treatment Want To Be In 'Control' 59
   Jason's Story 60
   Jovon's Story 63
   Shanika's Story 64
   Armando's Story... 67
   Azuka's Story 68
5. Individual Counseling: The First Line Of Offense In
   Working With Youths... 71
   Confronting Inconsistencies And Connecting Dots 76
   Stanley's Story 80
   Healing Emotional Injuries... 85
   Stanley's Story Continued 88
   Group Counseling For Youths: How It Works................... 102
   Gibson House Experience.. 104

J.C. Model 107
James' Story 109
6. The Eclectic Grill 112
Gestalt Approach 115
Alternate Treatment Approaches 125
Rational-Emotive Approach 133
Solution Focused Therapy 141

About The Author 163

PREFACE

The scourges of drug abuse manifest itself all around the world, from the Far East to the Western shores of the global hemisphere. Licit and illicit drug abuse erodes the fabric of every society in which it sprouts. In deed, once the seeds of drug abuse germinate on any national soil, it immediately pre-empts the social, economic, psychological, spiritual, and medical life of the indulgent. Along with that, comes the gradual and progressive chipping of the cement that binds the drug abusers community. Drug abuse in this book includes alcoholism. Drug abuse is not a new phenomenon. Cocaine abuse in the United States "began during the mid-1880s, reached a peak between 1900 and 1915, and then went into a period of sustained decline," (Spillane, 1998). Over the years, the damages associated with drug abuse to society gained precedence among societal social and medical problems. In 1969, Senator Harold Hughes (former Governor of Iowa State) was selected to chair the Senate Subcommittee on Alcoholism and Narcotics. The Comprehensive Alcoholism Prevention and Treatment Act of 1970 was signed into law by President Richard Nixon, following an extensive public hearing that included the testimony of Bill Wilson (co-founder of Alcoholics Anonymous). This statute, which came to be known as the Hughes Act, followed the Cooperative Commission's recommendations by creating a National Institute on Alcohol Abuse and Alcoholism, NIAAA, (White, 1998). According to White, the rise in youthful poly-drug abuse – and concern about drug use among soldiers in Vietnam – reached a political boiling point in 1971, forcing president Richard Nixon to declare drug abuse "America's Public Enemy Number One." Alongside the NIAAA was the creation of the Drug Abuse Treatment Act of 1972 that lead to the establishment of the National Institute on Drug Abuse (NIDA). The above mentioned Acts were instrumental in funding treatment, research, and education programs at an attempt to find a "cure" for drug abuse.

Drug abuse treatment targeted adults during its early inception. Adults needed treatment because drug abuse leads to dysfunction in social, family and work milieu. This, in turn, stymied adult productivity and thereby, caused recognizable problems to families and society at large. Drug abuse was perceived as a moral or social problem. As a result, early treatment consisted of asylum or incarceration. Medical treatment centered on eradicating the physiological symptoms of drug abuse such as delirium tremens associated with alcoholism or physical pain and diarrhea from opiate withdrawal. Even psychotic behavior from stimulant drug withdrawal was treated, rather than the underlying causes behind these symptoms. Psychologists and Psychiatrists spent valuable hours postulating theories on addictive personality type concepts in an attempt to treat drug abuse. In June 1935, the first AA group was formed in Akron, Ohio, during a talk between a New York stockbroker, Bill Wilson, and an Akron physician, Dr. Bob, (Alcoholics Anonymous, 1939). AA shed more light on drug abuse treatment when it introduced the concept of alcoholism as consisting of an allergy of the body and an obsession of the mind by emphasizing alcoholism to be a disease rather than a social problem. The establishment of the NIDA and the subsequent availability of funds for research led to more improvement in drug abuse treatment protocol. In fact, the last two decades have shown marked advances in research aimed at understanding the bio-psychogenics of addiction. Technology has added more dimensions to addiction studies through facilitation of more in-depth knowledge of pharmacology, neuroscience, and genetics. The more we understand addiction, the better we get at treating it. Contemporary addiction treatment emphasizes eclectic approach.

Addiction treatment is not a one-size fit all venture. Many adults who go to treatment do so because of one of three reasons: 1. They are forced to get treatment by the legal or family system, 2. They have sustained serious health problem because of addiction and death is imminent, or 3. They reached very low bottom in life, which precipitates a spiritual experience of some sort. The unique feature of any one of those reasons is that the adult will either seek treatment or face a more serious consequence. This realization ignites some level of willingness to enter treatment, even if it is mere lip service at the beginning. On the contrary, adolescents and youths often times lack the logical connection between substance abuse and adverse consequences arising from substance abuse. This obvious gap in logical sequencing deters willingness in adolescents and youths to seek treatment. By implication, this very aberration hardens the wall of denial about substance use and abuse among adolescents and youths, thereby making this population resistant to treatment.

Mini stories from real life clinical settings are used in this book to epitomize the severity of denial among youths in treatment. Names have been changed to protect clients whose lives have long been changed for the better. Other stories are full accounts of different kinds of street education and socialization that imbibe core values in our youths. These core values, even though may become self-defeating in the future, offer immediate protection against logical connection between substance use and abuse and consequences. They also offer coping skills to youths that have been verbally or physically abused, emotionally injured due to divorce, guilty by association with the wrong peers in school, neglected by parents, or victims of socio-economic ineptitude. These core values in question are rather generational than ethnic or racially targeted. In fact, most youths in substance abuse treatment irrespective of race or state of origin seem to have graduated from some legendary school of street survival academy. Their defense mechanisms, layered walls of denial and confrontational strategies are mostly identical.

Emphasis has deliberately been placed on working with marijuana-impaired youths because marijuana inflicts damage over a longer period of time. It also opens up doors to other hard drugs. Chapter one begins with a vignette to illustrate the progressive nature of marijuana addiction. The rather slow onset of consequences of marijuana abuse, coupled with its gateway properties, makes it a clinical puzzle. Working with marijuana abusing youths requires special skills. As you will see from flipping through this book various styles are used to confront irrational beliefs in marijuana abusing youths. Some techniques are differently familiar, yet others are completely unorthodox. In emphasizing novelty, many clinicians ignore old practices. Attempts have been made to strike a balance between powerful new ways of working with youths in treatment and classic research in psychotherapy. Classic researches in social psychology and psychology (e.g., implicit personality theory, rationalization trap, cognitive theory, gestalt, rational- emotive, and solution focused theories) have been credited for their role in understanding and treating youths. Some individual case studies are described in more detail to highlight the progressive nature of addiction and the beautiful transformation that occurs when youths can finally make the connection between substance abuse and overall progress in life.

ACKNOWLEDGEMENTS

I am indebted to my wife, Stephanie, and children (Kyle and Klyde), for their invaluable support while writing this book (especially for their love, patience and understanding, even when the hour was three o'clock in the morning and the computer chair was squeaking louder than life). Many thanks to my mentor and friend, Dr. Darryl Inaba, whose insatiable urge to uncover more facts about addiction and whose years of clinical experience are second to none. My gratitude is extended to my clients and trainees at Inland Empire Job Corps without whose practical experience in substance abuse and teachings this book would not have been possible. Thanks to Jeannie Broadus-Castillo for her gentle but persistent prodding and for allowing me unparalleled latitude in the use of eclecticism in the Job Corps youth treatment program. I am delighted to acknowledge the general contribution of my teacher and friend Dr. Donald Nessman, most notably his emphasis on the role of ego syntonism in working with youths. Special thanks to my colleagues at the annual School of Alcoholism and Chemical Dependency, University of Salt Lake City, Utah. No book can be written and published without the help of a great many people working with the author behind the scene, and this book is no exception. Thanks to the following people for their direct and indirect contribution in compiling this book:

Ejikay Jamelle Freeman Wachuku, DBCC, Daytona Beach
Sonnia (Nia) Adah Jamina Wachuku, University of Florida, Gainesville
Joan Harter, San Bernardino Valley College
Bernnie Breining, Breining Institute
Dr. Schubert Sapien, Fort Worth, TX

CHAPTER ONE

INTRODUCTION: THIS ADDICTION THING

In 1975, Ashley graduated from high school. During prom that year, she tried marijuana for the very first time. Her mom had told her about drugs. Her mom had also admitted that she and her stepfather had experimented with marijuana during their youth. However, Ashley's mom had cautioned that using drugs habitually would amount to a waist of productive life. She reminded Ashley that she and her stepfather were successful upper income class parents because they chose to not over indulge in the drug culture. This family moment set the pace for Ashley's drug-free secondary school years until prom night. Ashley's biological father had left her mom when she was three years old. She realized her stepfather was not her real father when she was eight years old. While in the fifth grade Ashley began to feel like her stepfather favored her younger sister and two brothers more. She had everything a child would want; yet the perception of favoritism from her stepfather bothered her. She lived with a slight resentment towards her stepfather throughout her high school years.

Ashley had an ambiguous perception of marijuana on that prom night experiment. But she did it again during the month following high school graduation. Then she did it again. And again. Suddenly, she cared less if her stepfather was partial or not towards her sister and brothers. She took her recreation drug use to college where she met other girls who also smoked marijuana. She graduated from high school with a C average grade. Ironically, while in college, she maintained more than a three-point average. She became philosophical and often told her friends she studied better and got better grades under the influence of marijuana. She also started drinking frequently at weekend parties with her friends. She graduated from college with over three-point average. She went to graduate school and continued her drug and alcohol life style. This time she graduated with a much higher GPA, missing four-point average by scoring a B in only one of her many graduate courses.

1

This, once again, confirmed her mythical prowess in the use of marijuana.

Ashley met an interesting male friend in graduate school. Shortly after graduation, they got married. Life was good for about six month after marriage. They both had good jobs and lived in the nice side of the city. In time Ashley became more interested in her marijuana smoking, preferring to stay in door than do outdoor recreation activity with her husband. As time passed, she drank more. She became argumentative and irate with her husband. She drank and smoked more, if her husband constructively criticized her. She told her husband time and time that marijuana was not addictive and that she will stop smoking it when she was ready. One night Ashley left with her female college-days friend to a party without her husband. At 2:30am that morning she called her husband from the county jailhouse to pick her up. She had had so much to drink that she was driving on the opposite side of a one-way street. A few months after that incident (few days away from her one year wedding anniversary) her husband divorced her.

The divorce dealt a blow to her career. She needed her drink and marijuana cigarette to get ready for work in the morning. And more drink at lunchtime. And then more drink after work on her way home. She loved to stop by the bar (happy hour) after work. She quickly became very friendly with the guys at the bar. She even knew the bar tenders by name. Later that year she was fired from her job. The year was now 1986, eleven years after that prom night marijuana experiment. While unemployed she met some friends who had some bright ideas on how to make lots of money in a very short time. Ashley was interested. The idea was to buy a kilogram of cocaine, split it four ways and distribute to four standby buyers who had the money to buy. She contributed half the money for the purchase ($5,500) from her savings. Ashley was to pick up the merchandize from an adjoining city. She flew in and out of the adjoining city, unnoticed, with a kilogram of cocaine. On return, her associates took their half of the product, told Ashley the buyers will pick up her portion the next morning at a nearby Denny's restaurant and left. She went to the restaurant as scheduled the next day with half a kilo of cocaine, but there were no buyers. She came back home somewhat confused about what to do with half a kilo of cocaine. She had no clue what the legal consequence of that much of cocaine would be.

Suddenly, eureka! She knew what to do. She went to the bar and shared her new business venture with some female associates in the hope they may know buyers. It was a marvel idea, except the two females she talked to use cocaine. They followed her home to sample the product and were stunned to know that Ashley had 97% pure cocaine crystal. They quickly convinced her to try her own product, so she will know what she was selling. Reluctantly, she did. She did not know what to expect in terms of the drug effect on her. All she remembered from that first experience with cocaine was that she was talkative and free spirited. She enjoyed intellectual discuss, naturally, so she became the center of attraction, at least in her mind. Another immediate effect cocaine had on her, she recalled, was a strange sexual arousal. One of the two female she brought home from the bar took care of Ashley sexual urge. At the end of the day, no cocaine was sold. She had become permissive to two new ventures: snorted cocaine and had sex with a female. Needless to mention that the two bar associates spent the night in her apartment and would stay with her for the next several days, doing the same thing over and over: get high, get drunk, and have sex. In a few days another friend joined the click. This one said she knew how to convert the cocaine hydrochloride to crack cocaine, which she said was more in demand. After two days of frustrating experimentation trying to cook up crack cocaine, half the product was wasted to no avail. A buyer was finally found who surprisingly paid Ashley $5,000 dollars, despite the waste. By now, Ashley had had enough. She decided to get away from it all.

She heard her cousin was moving west to stay with her sister, she made a spontaneous decision to leave town and start a new life. Her cousin had also been exposed to cocaine earlier and was also remotely getting away to start a new life. Together they set out to travel across the land from the east coast to the west coast. A two-day stop over in New Orleans triggered a resurgence of the cocaine party. They arrived in California and discovered cocaine was more readily available than it was back east, so the party continued. They found jobs and moved into an apartment together. This was the summer of 1987. By December the same year, they were evicted from their apartment. In early 1988, Ashley was arrested for assaulting her ex-boy friend with a deadly weapon over cocaine. Two weeks before the fight, she had called her ex-boy friend from back east out of loneliness. He had also fallen victim to cocaine habit, unbeknown to Ashley. He quickly volunteered to visit Ashley during that phone conversation in the hope that he too will escape from cocaine habit. On arrival to California, his and her cocaine usage exacerbated. By the summer of 1988, exactly one year after Ashley arrived in California, she was unable to keep a job. She began selling all her valuables to support her rapidly growing cocaine habit. When cocaine was not available, she used methamphetamine or phencyclidine. She charged her credit cards over reasonable limit and continued to charge them until the cards were cancelled. She was at some point arrested for writing NSF checks. She became completely homeless and lived with one associate after another, leaving a trail of burnt bridges. During these desperate moments she once again had one of her intellectual insight – she could sell cocaine like she once did back east and salvage her homeless status. So, she filed for unemployment and invested her first payment on cocaine sales. Within a short period of time she had established her presence in the petty dealers cocaine market. Life could not have been better. She could use all the cocaine she wanted, make a living and be responsibility free.

In 1990, fifteen years after that prom night experiment with marijuana, Ashley was arrested by the narcotic vice squad for possession of cocaine with intent to sell. The bail was high. Somehow, luck was on her side. After two weeks in county jail, she was released on her own recognizance because she did not have a prior case involving drugs. In the next eighteen months, Ashley trailed several minor arrests: failure to appears, riding in stolen vehicle, possession of drugs, etc. In 1991 she plea-bargained and was sentenced to ninety days in jail for the 1990 possession case. After she served her time, she became extremely cautious about dealing drugs. First, she became her own best customer; second, after she got out of jail, she had conned fellow petty dealers to loan her capital to re-enter the trade. She did not pay back any of them. She feared retribution and went underground. It was during this time that self-pity got the best of her. As time went by, it got harder for her to sustain her habits. She feared going back to jail. Finally, she made a decision to seek treatment.

March 1992, sixteen years after that prom night experiment with marijuana, Ashley walked into the author's office with a plastic shopping bag containing no more than three pieces of clothing and possibly one underwear (her entire wardrobe), looking for housing assistance with no money whatsoever. She had just completed ninety days of treatment in a social model residential treatment facility and was handed a piece of paper with the author's business address for housing/aftercare treatment assistance. She looked timid and scared. Her gaze seems to focus on some distant remote point far beyond the author as she asked, "Is this the sober living place?" Please sit down, she was ordered. Her long curly hair lay in lumps over her shoulders. Yet, wretched and haggard as she looked that morning, an uncanny aura of beauty radiated around her. It was noticeable that she had lived two lives in the immediate past. She began telling her seemingly life-long story of addiction before the author handed her a rental application form. "My name is Ashley, I am an addict. I am ninety days clean and sober…" There was an air of confidence in her voice when she said 'clean and sober.'

Names have been changed to protect the identities of all the clients whose stories have been told in this book. Ashley has long undergone complete rehabilitation, including vocational rehabilitation. She obtained another master's degree in social work and now runs one of the finest treatment centers for women with children. Ironically, she was invited to discuss the possible inclusion of her story in this publication in March 2002, ten years after she walked into the author's office with a plastic shopping bag. This time she walked in with a fine leather handbag. That tattered aura of beauty which radiated around her, ten years ago, was now a solid physical beauty imprinted in her gait and her every being. "Ok, my name is Ashley, I am an addict. I am ninety days clean and sober," she joked. When she smiled, a heavenly surge of hope spilt over the author's office. For every successful recovery story such as Ashley, many ended in utter hopelessness or perpetual acceptance of failure. Others amalgamated to complete dual diagnosis (substance abuse induced mental illness) condition. Yet, others ended in jails, institutions or death.

Ashley's story exemplifies the progressive nature of addiction. She had experimented with marijuana, experienced euphoria, and possibly a euphoric recall, which made her want to recapture that first time feeling, thereby priming her brain to develop tolerance for marijuana. Once she started enjoying the effects of marijuana, it opened the door for yet another gateway drug – alcohol. In time it culminated to poly-substance abuse. However, this story is more than a simple linear progression of drug use and abuse. Implicit in the story are other elements that characterize addiction. Addiction consists of genetic, environmental, psychological, physiological and socio-cultural aspects. We mentioned at the on set of this story that Ashley's parents had experimented with marijuana. We did not have full knowledge of her parent's involvement, nor did we trace back to her grand parents to determine if there is an addictive gene in the family. What we do know is that Ashley found herself in an environment where marijuana was readily available on prom night. We also know that she had a deep-seated resentment toward her stepfather for favoritism to her stepsister. This psychological or emotional injury became soothed, once she smoked marijuana. She quickly became physiologically dependent on marijuana the more she used it to process her feelings of inadequacy and insecurity in the family. Further, during and after college, she was in the mist of friends who shared her drug use lifestyle, which strongly predisposed her to the socio-cultural aspects of addiction. We shall fully explore these various aspects of addiction in chapter two.

The author observes that over the years working with youths, childhood emotional injury predominantly underlies most cases of addiction among youths. Almost every child experiences some form of mishap or psychological disappointment during late childhood or early adolescence period. Some are severe and others are mild. How each case is treated determines whether the child sustains injury or not. Most families tend to identify feelings of inadequacy, insecurity, low self worth, etc, within their children and appropriately address these issues. Other times, these issues go un-noticed and emanate as shyness, poor grades in school, negative attention, defiant behavior, to mention but a few. In other instances, abuse (physical, verbal or psychological) preempts emotional or psychological injury among youths. This underlying condition predisposes many youth to addiction. Most substances of abuse, including alcohol, have therapeutic properties when it comes to dealing with emotional injuries. A mentor once said: "There is no problem, no matter how severe, that drinking a full glass of Jack Daniel would not solve, at least temporarily." Many youths say they use marijuana because it helps them deal with stress in schools or families. Some adults agree alcohol helps them cope with stress. Excessive reliance on psychoactive substances as problems solvers may lead to addiction. This premise does not discount the genetic implications of addiction as evident in chapter two.

CHAPTER TWO

ADDICTION: DISEASE OR SOCIAL MALADJUSTMENT?

The debate on whether addiction is a disease or social problem has spanned over two centuries. Alan Leshner, Director of the National Institute on Drug Abuse (NIDA), noted during an interview with Professional Counselor Magazine in 1998 "We've come to learn that, at its core, addiction is a brain disease; but it's a brain disease that has imbedded in it, behavioral and social aspects. Those aspects require that we use sophisticated behavioral treatment techniques as an integral part of drug treatment." Those who see addiction as a social maladjustment tend to favor incarceration as the preferred treatment method. By contrast, social or medical model treatment is highly recommended by those who see addiction as a biological problem. Leshner warned that the mind-body problem is over. You don't have a separate mind and a separate body, so you have to see addiction as a truly bio-behavioral illness…They work together…It's important in treatment not to pit biology against behavior. We know that the individual's motivation can influence the course of treatment, but that doesn't mean that the individual's biology is uninvolved. The fact that it's a disease does not mean that you can't do something about it. We can do something about obesity, which is a disease; hypertension, which is a disease; stress, which is a disease, (Professional Counselor, p.39, October 1998).

William L. White (Counselor, October 2000) contends, "The debate over the disease concept of addiction is not a meaningless intellectual exercise. Any framework for understanding alcohol and other drug (AOD) problems exerts a profound influence on the lives of individuals, families, social institutions and communities." White asserts that the disease concept dates back to civilizations of ancient Egypt and Greece, and that calls for state-sponsored treatment continued through the centuries before the first Europeans migration to America. He traces the history of the disease concept back to the work of Anthony Benzet, social reformer, in 1774. Ten years later in

1784, Benjamin Rush's *Inquiry into the Effects of Ardent Spirits on the Human Mind and body* described "persons addicted to ardent spirits" as suffering from "odious disease induced by a vice," according to White. As the disease concept grew, so did treatment. Early treatment was varied and sometimes cruel. Samuel Woodward, a prominent physician, recommended the creation of special asylum for the treatment of inebriates in the 1830s, White noted. He further added that Woodward described how intemperance was a "physical disease, which preys upon (the drunkard's) health and spirits…making him a willing slave to his appetite." Heredity was also highlighted as a causative factor in chronic drunkenness. Prior to Woodward's work, Dr. William Sweetser argued in 1829 that intemperance directly or indirectly created a "morbid alteration" in nearly all major structures and functions of the human body, (Counselor, p.48, October 2000). Sweetser's study reflects the dichotomy that biases modern concern of addiction as a disease. According to White, Sweetser cautions:

> Now that (intemperance) becomes a disease no one doubts, but then it is a disease produced and maintained by voluntary acts, which is a very different thing from a disease with which providence inflicts us…I feel convinced that should the opinion ever prevail that intemperance is a disease like fever, mania, etc., and no moral turpitude be affixed to it, drunkenness, if possible, will spread itself even to a more alarming extent than at present.

Early alcoholic mutual aid societies like the Washingtonians from which Alcoholics Anonymous originated recognized alcoholism as a disease. However, the disease concept did not grow without resistance. Dr. C.W. Earle of Chicago wrote: "It is becoming altogether too customary in these days to speak of vice as disease…That the responsibility of taking the opium or whiskey…is to be excused and called a disease, I am not willing for one moment to admit, and I propose to fight this pernicious doctrine as long as is necessary," (Counselor, p.49, 2000). Dr. Robert Harris of Franklin

Reformatory for Inebriates in Philadelphia was equally opposed to the disease concept. In 1874 he stated the position of his institution on the disease concept: "As we do not, either in name or management, recognize drunkenness as the effect of a diseased impulse; but regard it as a habit, sin, and crime, we do not speak of cases being cured in a hospital, but 'reformed'," (ibid). White contends that the demedicalization of addiction rose in the wake of alcohol and drug prohibition movements. The disease concept returned with revamping of the old Washingtonian movement under the auspices of Bill Wilson and Dr. Bob in 1935. This time, the concept was to undergo a more scientific scrutiny. We shall examine in more details the contemporary definition of addiction and research in favor of the disease concept.

WHAT IS ADDICTION?

Addiction is a compulsive obsessive behavior disorder that has baffled scholars and practitioners in the field of social work, psychiatry, psychology and medicine. Indeed, addiction disorder poses a challenge to society at large. Whenever addictive disorder is mentioned, substance dependence is what comes to mind, although addictive disorder generally encompasses substance dependence. The Diagnostic and Statistical Manual (DSM-IV) diagnostic criteria for substance dependence states that three of the following conditions must be present in a 12- month period in other for substance dependence to occur:

- Taken in large amount over time than intended
- Desire or unsuccessful effort to control or cut down
- Great deal of time spent in obtaining, using, or recovering from effects of use
- Social, occupational, recreational activities given up because of use
- Continued use despite social, legal, medical, psychological, other problems
- Tolerance
- Withdrawal

The Manual cautions that criteria can be met without tolerance or withdrawal and, conversely, tolerance and withdrawal, do not meet criteria. Traditionally, stereotypical conception of addictive disorder centers on alcohol and narcotics addiction. In recent times, addictive disorder has expanded its realm to include other areas of behavior, vis-à-vis: gambling, running, shopping, sex and over-eating, to mention but a few. Several theories have been postulated in search of a meaningful understanding of addictive disorder. The author explores some of these theories organized into sections on genetic theories, inherited mechanisms that cause or predispose people to be addicted; metabolic theories, biological or cellular adaptation to chronic exposure to drugs; and cultural genetic theories, based on racial inheritance. A growing trend in the quest to understand addictive disorder is the classification of addictive disorder as a disease. This concept recognizes that alcoholism is a primary addictive response to alcohol in a biologically susceptible drinker, regardless of character and personality, or of cultural or psychosocial influences. Researchers have identified this concept as the biogenic model. The opposite end of the spectrum of the disease concept is based on the belief that alcoholism is a symptom or consequence of an underlying character defect, a self-destructive response to psychological and social problems, and that it is a learned behavior. This is the psychogenics model. The two models are sometimes treated as mutually exclusive. The failed attempts at compromise highlights the fact that the exact pathophysiology of addiction is not known. In trying to understand the matrix of addictive disorder, several conflicting notions have been advanced. Some see addiction as caused by abnormal or different receptors for neurotransmitters such as dopamine or serotonin, different neuroanatomical connections, or different chemical response to addictive drugs. Yet, others see addiction as a dispositional disease model, but also list moral temperance, spiritual, educational, social, characterologic, biologic, conditioning, socio-cultural, and general system, etc.

Putting addiction disorder in a nomenclature is difficult and that makes it harder to understand addiction. If we knew for sure that a defective gene, say the CYP2A6 enzyme is the cause of addiction, then we can easily understand the disease concept. It will be easily accepted that an addict suffers from CYP2A6 deficiency disease. Such is hardly the case. Most people have an erroneous view of disease as something that invades or attacks your good health; an innocent victim attacked by a "perpetrator" over whom he or she has no control. Such skewed view of addiction alienates the psychosocial and environmental argument in favor of addictive disorder. The idea of disease does not work well for addiction. In addiction, the person participates in or causes many of their own problems by their behavior. Some scholars agree that there appears to be a hereditary genetic component to addiction. What is inherited, they say, is the potential for addiction and not the disease.

Implicitly, the disease model of addiction gained a new popularity when the publication *Alcoholics Anonymous* (1939) began peddling the idea of the alcoholic as a person who from birth was destined to be unable to control her/his drinking. The argument was advanced that such a person suffers from an allergy of the body, which subjects the person to an inexorable path to intoxication and to an eventual diseased state. Coupled with that notion is the 'obsession of the mind' component to the allergy. The said obsession is uncanny by nature and over-powers the afflicted to pursue the urge to imbibe in alcohol drinking with a perpetual inability to refrain from the overwhelming urge. With the transfer of the crucial mechanism from the substance (alcohol) to the consumer, A.A. presented the view that the compulsion to drink was biologically programmed and thus inevitably characterized drinking by alcoholics. Seemingly unsystematic as the A.A. concept may have appeared, patients and family alike benefit from understanding the A.A. position. The understanding helps the patient to have less shame and guilt and to begin a process of accepting help. The family, in turn, benefits by decreasing anger and frustration, and they begin to support healthy rehabilitative activities for the patient and themselves. The concept offers a win-win approach to alcoholism treatment. Beneficial as the A.A. concept may seem, no biological mechanism has been found to support the claim of loss of control that A.A. advances. Even the most severely alcoholic individual "clearly demonstrates positive source of control over drinking behavior…extreme drunkenness cannot be accounted for on the basis of some internally located inability to stop" (Heather and Robertson 1981:122). Ironically, though, Heather and Robertson propose exceptions to their own analysis by asserting "some problem drinkers are born with physiological abnormality, either genetically transmitted or as a result of intrauterine factors, which make them react abnormally to alcohol from their first experience of it" (Heather and Robertson 1983: 141).

Empirical investigation of the A.A. implied disease concept revealed no basis for believing that alcoholics lost control of their drinking whenever they tasted alcohol (Marlatt et al., 1973; Merry, 1966; Paredes et al., 1973). Vaillant (1983) found that self-repots by A.A. members that they immediately succumbed to alcoholism the first time they drank were false and that severe drinking problems developed over periods of years and decades. The exceptions to this generalization were psychopaths whose drinking problems were components of overall abnormal lifestyle and behavior patterns from an early age. However, these kinds of alcoholics showed a greater tendency to outgrow alcoholism by moderating their drinking (Goodwin et al. 1971), indicating they also do not conform to a putative biological model. Prospective studies of those from alcoholic families also have failed to reveal early alcoholic drinking (Knop et al. 1984). Laboratory studies of drinking behavior of alcoholics did more than dispose the simplistic notion of a biologically based loss of control.

The work of Mello and Mendelson (1972), Nathan and Obrien (1971), and the Baltimore City Hospital group (Bigelow et al., 1974; Cohen et al., 1971) showed that alcoholic behavior could not be described in terms of an internal compulsion to drink, but rather that even alcoholics (while drinking) remained sensitive to environmental and cognitive inputs, realized the impact of reward and punishment, were aware of the presence of others around them and of their behavior, and drank to achieve a specific level of intoxication. For example, Mello and Mendelson (1972) found that alcoholics worked to accumulate enough experimental credits to be able to drink two or three days straight, even when they were already undergoing withdrawal from previous intoxication. Alcoholics observed by Bigelow et al. (1974) drank less when the experimenters forced them to leave a social area to consume their drinks in an isolated compartment. Many aspects of this laboratory portrait of the social, environmental and intentional elements in alcoholic imbibing correspond to the picture of problem drinking that was provided by the national survey conducted by Cahalan and his co-workers (Cahalan, 1972; Cahalan and Room, 1974; Clark and Cahalan, 1976).

Virtually from the start, research directed at the disease idea proved unfavorable. Aside from two useful scientific contributions from E.M. Jellinek – a phased symtomatology from alcoholism (Jellinek, 1952) and the prevalence estimation formula that bore his name (Jellinek, 1951) – alcohol science created more difficulties than support for this central idea. Whether it was Haggard's (1944) early empirical rejection of A.A.'s allergy hypothesis, Jackson's (1958) disconfirming analyses of the alcohol syndrome, Syme's (1957), negative review of the prospective of discerning an alcoholic proved hostile to the idea's various empirical test-point. Even the Supreme Court – in Powell v. Texas (Fingarette, 1970) – could not quite bring itself to ratify the disease concept when it got the opportunity in 1968.

GENETIC PREDISPOSITION TO ADDICTION

The foregoing research concerns on the disease concept of addiction culminated into further research at an attempt to uncover some form of genetic predisposition to addiction. Since A.A. had unintentionally prodded or aroused scientific curiosity with its disease theory of alcoholism, it is not surprising that early research to determine a genetic link to addiction was geared toward alcoholism. The early work of Jellinek, (1952), although not probing the genes directly, heralded further curiosity among scholars to uncover a genetic link to addiction. In the past decade, the number of researchers investigating the topic has tripled, along with the assumption that alcoholism is at least in part genetically caused. For example, the National Institute on Alcohol Abuse and Alcoholism published a pamphlet in 1985 titled "Alcoholism: An Inherited Disease." Kenneth Blum, a pharmacologist at the University of Texas Health Science Center, San Antonio, and Ernest Noble, a psychiatrist and biochemist at the UCLA Alcohol Research Center and a former director of the National Institute of Alcohol Abuse and Alcoholism, published a study in April 1990 in the Journal of American Medical Association linking alcoholism to hereditary.

The Blum-Noble team probed nine different genes, all hypothetically linked to alcoholism in the DNA of the brains they examined. They found that only the Al allele of the dopamine D2 receptor gene correlated significantly with the diagnosis of alcoholism in their subjects, according to Stanton Peele, The Atlanta Monthly, *Second Thoughts About a Gene for Alcoholism.* Media coverage claimed the JAMA study appeared to offer "strong new evidence" for the heritability of alcoholism. The Blum-Noble study *Alcoholism and the Addictive Brain* sought to demonstrate that alcoholism is not only a biogenic disease characterized by genetic anomalies, but also that a wide range of excessive behavior can be traced to a similar defect. In 1993, Joel Gelernter of Yale and his colleagues surveyed all the studies that examined the Blum-Noble allele and alcoholism. Discounting Blum and Noble's research, the combined results were that 18 percent of nonalcoholics, 18 percent of problem drinkers, and 18 percent of severe alcoholics all had the allele. There was simply no link between this gene and alcoholism. Unfortunately, Gallup polls continue to show that 90 percent of the American public believes alcoholism is a disease, and more than 60 percent think it may be inherited, said Peele.

Recent research on genetic mechanisms in alcoholism presupposes that the genetic transmission of alcoholism has been firmly established. Support for this idea has been provided by research, which found greater concordance rates in alcoholism for identical versus fraternal twins and on the greater influence of the biologic versus the adoptive family in the development of alcoholism among adoptees (Goodwin, 1979). For example, Goodwin et al. (1973) found that male adoptees with alcoholic parents were four times more likely to become alcoholics than those without, although there was no such relationship with alcohol misuse in adoptive parents. Bohman (1978) and Cadoret and Gath (1978) also found this significantly enhanced liability for alcoholism among adopted male offspring of alcoholics. Similarly, Schuckit et al. (1972) discovered that half-siblings with at least one alcoholic-biologic parent were far more likely to develop alcoholism than those without such a parent, no matter by whom they were raised. These studies did not pass without correspondingly disapproving research findings.

Further studies on the adopted twin research had strong implications that the inability to control drinking is not inherited. Subsequently, attempts were made to explore other theories of genetic predisposition. One such area is the process of alcohol metabolism in humans. Speculations about metabolic difference have a long history, and the metabolic process that has attracted perhaps the greatest interest recently has been the accumulation of acetaldehyde following drinking (Lieber, 1976; Milam and Ketcham, 1983). Schuckit and Rayses (1979) found that young men with familial history of alcoholism showed levels of acetaldehyde after drinking that were double the levels of those without such histories. Other metabolic processes that have traditionally been of interest have been the more rapid onset and peak experience of physiological reactions to alcohol, as in the visible flush typical of the drinking in Oriental populations.

Working from the opposite direction, Schuckit (1980, 1984b) has found the offspring of alcoholics to be less sensitive to their blood alcohol levels. This type of finding may indicate that those with a pedigree for alcoholism are not as aware of the onset of intoxication when they drink or that they have a greater tolerance for alcohol. Stanton Peele (1990) contend that the acetaldehyde hypothesis got strong play in the widely read book *Under the Influence*, by Jamea Milan and Katherine Ketcham, which was published in 1981. "Milam and Ketcham forcefully argued that acetaldehyde is a primary biological and genetic basis for alcoholism, which they claim is completely biologically determined," Peele wrote. The other area of heritability of alcoholism that attracted the attention of researchers is brain wave abnormality. Research in this area tends to purport that children of alcoholics inherit cognitive and neurological impairment. Henri Begleiter (1984), a psychiatrist at the Downstate Medical Center, in Brooklyn, contend that brain wave abnormalities were found among children of alcoholics who have never drunk alcohol.

Other studies show that children of alcoholic were deficient in test that measured coordination and intellectual abilities. Such cognitive and neurological impairment have frequently been found in alcoholic parents in perceptual-motor, memory and language-processing tasks (Tarter et al.1984), whereas adults with alcohol relatives did worse than those with no family alcoholism history in abstract problem solving, perceptual-motor tasks and to a lesser extent, verbal and learning-memory tests (Schaeffer et al., 1984). The discrepancies in the latter study held for those with familial alcoholism whether or not they themselves were alcoholics. Begleiter and co-workers (1984) found that brain-wave abnormalities that were similar to those measured in alcoholics appeared in young boys with alcoholic fathers who themselves had never been exposed to alcohol, Gabrielli et al. (1982) had found that a similar group of children showed greater fast (beta) wave activity than a group of controls.

RACIAL PREDISPOSITION TO ALCOHOLISM

Somehow identical twin research, metabolic differences, and brain wave abnormalities, failed to pinpoint a clear and definite explanation for the argument in favor of the genetics of addiction disorder predisposition theory. Researchers turned to another area of human coincidence or apparent co-relation – cultural genetic acquisition of alcoholism. The striking impetus in this area of research is the observation that people of certain national and/or racial origin tend to be more or less addicted to alcohol than others, thereby raising speculation that such co-relation may be the direct result of inherited gene. This observation goaded researches to explore why, for example, the Irish relatively drank more than others. Or, why the Native American and the Eskimo population have a high number of alcoholism cases. Yet, some researchers wonder why people of Asian origin tend to have lower alcoholism tendencies. Schuckit (1984) proposed that alcoholics inherit a different style of metabolizing alcohol, such as producing higher level of acetaldehyde due to drinking. The Asian population was known to inherit the hyper-responsive effect to alcohol. The hyper-metabolism to alcohol is characterized by a defective gene which makes it possible for Asians to respond to alcohol effect in a more rapid progression than it would on other races, thereby leading to a condition described as the

Oriental flush. As if to buttress this claim, Barnett (1955) examined police blotters in the Chinatown district of New York. He found that among 17,515 arrests recorded between 1933 and 1949, not one reported drunkenness in the charge.

On the contrary, Native American population and Eskimo group share the same so-called defective gene that hasten the onset of intoxication and a visible reddening from ingesting small amount of alcohol. Unlike the Asian population, the American Indians and Eskimo population gave very high incidence of alcohol abuse and alcoholism. This aberration leads to other speculations regarding racial genetic theory. In fact, Shkinlyk (1984) in his case study titled "A poison stronger than love" highlighted the contrast in alcohol effect on the Ojibwa Indian community in northwest Ontario. In this community, violent assault and suicide are so prevalent that only one in four die of natural cause or by accident. According to the study, in one year one-third of the children between five and fourteen were taken from their parents because the parents were unable to care for the children because of continuous drunkenness. This village was marked by "cycle of forced migration, economic dependence, loss of cultural identity, and breakdown in social networks" (Chance, 1985, p. 65) that underlay its self-destruction through alcohol.

GENETIC PREDESPOSITION TO OTHER DRUGS

As studies in alcohol addiction and predisposition continued, some research began investigating similar occurrence in other narcotic drugs. When most of the Vietnam Veterans who were addicted to heroin returned home and continued normal life without furthering their addiction, researchers began pondering over the underlying difference between narcotic and alcohol use. In fact, the idea that addiction was an inevitable consequence of narcotic use – even for some who had been previously dependent on drugs – prompted theorizing about inbred biological difference that produced differential susceptibility to narcotic addiction. Several pharmacologists posited that some drug users suffered a deficiency in endogenous opioid peptides, or endorphins, which made them particularly responsive to external infusion of narcotics (Goldstein,

1976; Snyder, 1977). Endorphin shortages as a potential causative factor in addiction also offered the possibility of accounting for other addictions and excessive behavior like alcoholism and overeating, that might affect endorphin levels (Weisz and Thompson, 1983).

Indeed, other pathological behaviors such as compulsive running were thought by some to be mediated by this same neurochemical system (Pargman and Baker, 1980). In recent times, clinical and biomedical investigators have began to explore genetic mechanisms for all addiction because of growing clinical awareness that approximately the same percentage of people become addicted to a range of psychoactive substances, including alcohol, valium, the narcotics and cocaine (McConnell, 1984; Peele, 1983). The first prominent example of genetic theory of addiction other than in the case of alcoholism arose from Dole and Nyswander's (1967) hypothesis that heroin addiction was a metabolic disease. For these researchers, incredibly high relapse rates for treated heroin addicts indicated a possible physiological basis for addiction, which transcended the active presence of the drug in the user's system. What this permanent or semi-permanent residue from chronic use might comprise was not clearly specified in the Dole-Nyswander's formulation. Meanwhile, this disease theory was confused by evidence not only that addiction occurred for a minority of those exposed to narcotics, but that addicts – especially those not in treatment – often did outgrow their drug habits (Maddux and Desmond, 1981; Waldorf, 1983) and that quite a few were subsequently able to use narcotic in a non-addictive fashion (Harding et al., 1980; Robin et al., 1974).

A 1997 study indicated that whether a person has a positive or negative sensation after smoking marijuana is heavily influenced by heredity. The study funded by the National Institute on Drug Abuse (NIDA), National Institute of Health, demonstrated that identical male twins were more likely than non-identical male to report similar responses to marijuana use, indicating a genetic basis for their sensation. Dr. Michael Lyons, Dr. Ming Tsuang, and colleagues at the Harvard Medical School in Boston, compared identical and fraternal twins of a series of questions in a detailed confidential interview of how "pleasant" or "unpleasant" they felt after smoking marijuana.

The identical twins answered similarly, while the fraternal twins did not. The results indicate that genes have a significant influence on individual pleasant or unpleasant responses to the effect of marijuana. A similar finding was made on caffeine in 1999. NBC News Archives reported that researchers at Virginia Commonwealth University studied nearly two thousand identical female twins, and they say that their gene influenced how much caffeine they drank and how likely they were to become addicted to caffeine. "From the perspective of a geneticist, does caffeine look dramatically different from nicotine, from ethanol, from cannabis? The answer is no. Pretty much the same," Dr. Kenneth Kendler said.

Another article published in the Environmental Health Perspective Volume, 106, Number 5, May 1998, indicated that "twin studies consistently indicate important genetic influence on multiple aspects of smoking behavior…In addition, genetic differences in nicotine receptors or nicotine metabolism might reasonably be hypothesized to play a role in smoking addiction." Another NBC News (1998) noted that "A team from the University of Toronto studied variations in the gene for an enzyme called CYP2A6. The body uses this particular enzyme in the liver to break down nicotine, the addictive component of cigarettes. They found that people with a common defect in the gene could only metabolize nicotine very slowly. This meant they were less likely to develop an addiction, and if they did smoke, they smoked fewer cigarettes than people without the fault." One twin study suggested that having a certain form of the gene makes it easier to kick the cigarette habit, or perhaps avoid getting hooked in the first place. "This is just one small piece of the puzzle of what influences smoking behavior," said psychologist Caryn Lerman, author of one of the studies, who is also the director of cancer genetics at the Lombardi Cancer Center of Georgetown University Medical Center in Washington. Science Daily Magazine, (1999), article stated that "researchers discovered that people carrying a particular version of the dopamine transporter gene (SLC6A3-9) are less likely to start smoking before the age of 16 and are more likely to be able to quit smoking if they start. Another Science Daily Magazine, (1998), news reported that "researchers from the University of Michigan Medical School asked female smokers, ex-smokers, and non-smokers about the sensations they felt when they tried smoking the first time. The smokers—especially the heavy smokers—were much more likely to say they experience pleasurable effects, such as a 'buzz' or relaxation."

Facts available indicate that many Americans believe in the predisposition to addiction theory for its obvious therapeutic value. More recently, the trend has extended to predisposition to behavioral addiction. Peele and Brodsky (1975) postulated that any powerful experience could form the object of an addiction for people predisposed by combinations of social and psychological factors. Their approach was anti-directional and rejected the deterministic force of inbred, biological, or other factors outside the realm of human consciousness and experience. Some predisposition to behavior theory suggest that addictive disorder tend to reciprocate into various range of other addiction whether it be behavioral or substance abuse. Smith (1981) posited the existence of an "addictive disease" to account for why so many of those who become addicted to one substance have prior histories of addiction to dissimilar substances. Working along the same line, Istvan and Matarazzo (1984) explored the possibilities both that these substances are "linked by reciprocal activation mechanisms" and may be linked by their "pharmacologically antagonistic…effects" (p.322).

In 1996, CNN News noted "New scientific research released Tuesday at a meeting in Chicago reveals that compulsive gambling may in fact be genetically founded." The news story identified the gene responsible for addictive gambling as the D-2 receptor. According to CNN News, in some people alcohol, drugs, sex, food or 'lots of gambling' can stimulate the D-2 receptor. The crux of the research was that compulsive gamblers share a gene that predisposes them to addictive behavior. The story cites Dr. David Comings of City of Hope National Medical Center as saying that "Environmental factors are important. It's a complex disorder. But genes also play a role and this is one of the genes." Attributing behavioral addiction to gene was taken one step forward when a former gynecologist sued his insurance company to collect disability benefits because he can't practice his specialty, according to a news story in The Courier Journal, October 1999. In 1998, the Kentucky Board of Medical

Licensure ordered Dr. Harold D Crall to stop practicing obstetrics and gynecology, go to work for the Department of Corrections and never to see female patients without a chaperone, following sexual misconduct charges. Dr. Crall filed suit in U.S. District Court against Provident Life & Accident Insurance Company, demanding $8,700 a month in disability payments in 1999. Dr. Charles F. Francke, a Louisville psychiatrist who diagnosed Crall with sexual addiction wrote: "There is no question in my mind, as with all addictions, a sexual addiction is a disease with a genetic predisposition." Compulsive over-eating leading to obesity has also been linked to genetic predisposition. A research study in the New England Journal of Medicine," An Adoption Study of Human Obesity," 1986, (volume 314: 193-198) indicated genetic predisposition to obesity. The idea of Genetic predisposition to obesity is not novel. Nisbett (1972) proposed an internal regulatory mechanism called set-point that is inherited or determined by parental or early childhood eating habit to be the cause of obesity. Nisbett's theory was that the hypothalamus was set to defend a specific body weight and that going below this weight stimulated a greater desire to eat.

All of the foregoing research presented evidence that there appears to be a genetic predisposition to addictive disorder. However, for any one research cited, myriads of opposing researches were equally advanced. To narrow the problem of addictive disorder purely to biogenic terms is do injustice to the field of substance abuse/behavioral science. Social, political, psychological, and general environmental factors all play key roles in addictive disorder. To isolate these environmental variables is to do disservice to social science and society at large. Such exclusionary approach to genetic formulations defies ample evidence that abound and deters future research. Interestingly enough, no findings from genetically oriented research have disputed the significance of behavioral, psychodynamic, existential and social-group factors in all the addictive disorder research. Schuckit (1984b), for example, announces, "that it is unlikely that there is a single cause for alcoholism that is both necessary and sufficient to produce the disorder. Peele (1980) importunes that "A successful addiction model must synthesize pharmacological, experimental, cultural, situational, and personality components in a fluid and seamless description of addictive motivation. It must account for why a drug is more addictive in one society than another, addictive for one individual and not another, and addictive for the same individual at one time and not another...The model must make sense out of the essentially similar behavior that takes place with all compulsive involvements. In addition, the model must adequately describe the cycle of increasing yet dysfunctional reliance on an involvement until the involvement overwhelms other reinforcements available to the individual.

There is need for research in the area of predisposition to addictive disorder. Current treatment approaches suffer a vicious cycle of recidivism. A genetic or socio-psycho-biogenic understanding of addiction disorder will offer much needed treatment implication to addictive disorder. Further, such understanding will enhance preventive measure as well as help in developing resiliency factors for the addiction prone individuals. On a more serious note, curative measures will be taken, given an adequate knowledge of the causes of addiction disorder. The University of Pittsburgh research team discovered a genetic sequence known as DRD5, which animal studies have linked to cocaine addiction, according to The Irish Independent, July 13, 1998. Dr. Michael Vanyukov, head of the genetic research team at the university's Center for Education and Drug Abuse Research, stated, "We hope to develop a measure of risk that would include both relevant genes and environment factors, and develop preventative measures that could offset even a high genetic predisposition to addiction." He added that "finding could lead to more sophisticated ways of assessing a person's risk to drug abuse." Dr. Jeffery Long of the National Institute of Health, speaking on CNN News, May 20, 1998, asserts, "even if the person did not become an alcoholic, it could be useful to know that they might transmit the gene." Mary Anne Rossing wrote in Environmental Health Perspective, Volume 105, Number 5, May 1998: A role of doperminergic or other genes in smoking cessation is of particular potential importance, as research in this area may lead to the identification of subgroups of individuals for whom pharmacologic cessation aids may be most effective.

BBC Online Network, June 24, 1998, reporting on the CYP2A6 nicotine metabolite enzyme noted: It was possible a pill or patch that blocked the enzyme could be developed to help people kick the smoking habit. Science Daily Magazine, January 26, 1999, reporting on the SLC6A3-9 gene quoted: with more of an understanding of the genetics of cigarette smoking behavior, we can develop more effective, targeted pharmacological psycho educational cessation strategies that will take these individual differences into account. Stanton Peele summed up treatment implications of genetic predisposition research in his review of Kenneth Blum's book *Alcohol and the Addictive Brain*: But if, as Blum claims, genetic discoveries will bring tremendous progress in fighting alcoholism, prayer will no longer be the primary treatment for the disease. Alcoholics might even be able to drink normally once their flawed addictive genes are modified (a futuristic procedure Blum describes) or when the chemical imbalance that is the cause is remedied by drug therapy. This inherent conflict between A.A. and medical approaches leads Blum and Payne, on the one hand, to attack those who question the disease theory and think "alcoholism can be arrested, and often cured," and, on the other, to predict that "the next forty years will bring cures…for compulsive disease such as alcoholism, drug addiction, and food disorders."

As has been noted earlier in this paper, there are inherent shortcomings to genetic predisposition research. Findings have not been consistent with the expected outcome. Nor has research findings been able to apply to different racial, social and gender classifications. Indeed, some have wondered if racial genome research is a fact or fiction.

Peele (1995) observed "the same DNA can function in more than one gene, making the concept of individual genes something of a convenient fiction. The mystery of how these genes, and the chemistry underlying them, cause specific traits and disease is a convoluted one." All studies have found that it is sons and not daughters who most often inherit the risk of alcoholism (Cloninger et al. 1978). One wonders, under what special circumstance can the genetic mappings explain this sex linkage? The fact that both the American Indians and the Asian population studied in New York have the same defective gene, yet they suffer bipolar effects of the same genetic marker raises serious research questions.

In the interest of all fairness, it is safe to assume that we do not have all the answers to genetic predisposition to addiction. The habitability of identical twin research is not based on human genome splicing, but instead on concordance rate. Those findings isolate the environmental and social forces at play. In the twin study implicating genetic predisposition to marijuana smoking, Dr. Lyons warned that "The specific genes involved could not be identified from this study, but it is speculated they are those involved in the brain's reward system." Ken Kidd, a Yale University geneticist who studied genetic markers used by researchers in the nicotine twin study cited earlier in this paper, criticized the design of the studies: I do not accept their conclusions, he said. Other research centered on brain wave scanning and high concordance rate of alcoholism among children of alcoholics has also been questioned. Children of alcoholics are said to inherit abnormal brain wave and other cognitive or neurological impairments, but Henri Begleiti (1984) has found such abnormalities in alcoholics' sons who have never drunk alcohol.

Other research teams have found different abnormalities in the brain-wave pattern of different groups of alcoholics and children of alcoholics. Even Schuckit finds the result of these researches inconsistent. In one of his researches, using subjects who on average had completed more than three years of college, he found no cognitive impairments among children of alcoholics. There is no doubt that the environment and social acceptability of drinking patterns play a role in alcoholism and other addictive disorder. In society where gambling is not legal or where gambling is not a way of life, it is unlikely that compulsive gambling will be a problem. Alcoholism is relatively very low among Moslems, because their religion forbids imbibing. Research indicates that people in lower socio-economic class tend to have more drinking problem. The Irish who tend to socially accept their plight as heavy drinkers may have more problems with alcoholism. Other small-scale research indicate that low income neighborhood where alcohol is sold at every corner of the city block have more drinking in those areas. All of these facts point to the conclusion that addictive disorder is a socio-econoculturogenic disorder. Robert Cloninger contend that "The demonstration of the critical importance of sociocultural influences in most alcoholics suggest that major changes in social attitudes about drinking styles can change dramatically the prevalence of alcohol abuse, regardless of genetic predisposition."

Research findings have a lead-on effect on the public and can very easily be misconstrued. Most studies that proclaim genetic predisposition usually have short- comings or research limitations hidden at the bottom of the findings. The mass media have a tendency to publicize the major premises of a study and ignore the limitations. The general public is lead on to believe those studies as absolutes. A recent study on the front page of The Sun, San Bernardino City newspaper claimed there might be medicinal value to nicotine. The way the headline was worded, it was easy for one to assume that smoking cigarettes would cure Alzheimer and other diseases. Some researches on addictive disorder are done on animals. Humans may react differently to some of these researches. Peele cautions: "Rats can be bred to drink large quantities of alcohol. But rats do not have values and culture that contravene the urge to drink excessively. While human beings clearly differ in how their bodies process and respond to alcohol, these differences do not translate into alcoholism independent of individual needs, opinions, and values. Someone who has a strong reaction to alcohol, or who cannot sense when he or she has had too much to drink, may just as easily choose habitually to stop after one or two drinks as to become intoxicated."

SOCIO-PSYCHOLOGY OF YOUTH MARIJUANA ADDICTION

There is an on-going rhetorical debate in the field of addiction study, namely: Nature vs. Nurture. Proponents of nature argue that addiction is a disease of the brain, mind and body. They argue that certain people are predisposed to becoming addicted either due to certain defective genes in their body or due to heritable traits that make them susceptible to addiction. On the other hand, opponents of the nature debate simply assert that over-indulgence in any substance use is a conscious decision. They maintain that a disease is something an innocent victim contracts or become afflicted with. They argue that conversely, addiction is a habit that the indulgent makes a conscious decision to involve in and therefore cannot fall in the same realm as a disease. They argue that addiction develops as a direct result of the social environment. A closer look at the social and psychological dynamics behind youth marijuana addiction may reveal some interesting aspects of addiction. Darryl S. Inaba and William E. Cohen (1989) contend that addiction occurs as the body adapts to drug toxicity on biological and cellular levels. They assert that sufficient amounts of drugs are ingested over time, which results in body and brain cell changes. These changes include: *tolerance* – an increasing need to escalate the drug dosage in order to maintain the euphoric high, a reaction that is partially due to liver function; *tissue dependence* – the development of cell alterations, which now cause the body to depend upon the drug to maintain balance; *withdrawal syndrome* – the occurrence of physical signs and symptoms of cessation (for example, depression, lethargy, sleeping problems, etc., when the drug is withdrawn); *psychic dependence* – a reliance on brain chemistry changes caused by usage, for example, altered states of consciousness and distortions of perception, which allows the user to avoid unpleasant realities, compensates for genetically missing brain reward hormones, and/or become dependent on the mesmerizing effects of the drug's positive reinforcement actions.

Youth marijuana addiction goes beyond Inaba and Cohen's simplistic academic view of addiction. There is an intricate psychological and social interplay that preempts the onset of youth marijuana addiction. After all, a youth may be predisposed to addiction or may have defective neurological enzymes, but unless the youth actually smokes marijuana, addiction may never ensue. Fifteen years of clinical experience working with youths reveals that peer pressure is the single most important factor in youth marijuana addiction. One pragmatic clinical tool that helped youths learn resistance skills to negative peer pressure was to have youths reenact a successful negative peer pressure. This exercise called for youths to role-play how they were able to convince other non-marijuana using youths to use drugs. Youths were asked to remember every minute details. Later, each step was carefully examined and a resistance skill was applied in various stages of the peer pressure to counteract and

27

diffuse the pressure. During this exercise, it became clear that there were several stages of change in the final decision to use marijuana by the unsuspecting "innocent" youth who had never tried marijuana before. Indeed, according to the youths, few kids smoked marijuana the first time they were confronted or peer pressured. Prochaska and DiClemente postulate that clients undergo six stages of change in the process of accepting treatment. Those same stages which send clients to treatment -1. Pre-contemplation, 2. Contemplation, 3. Preparation, 4. Action, 5. Maintenance, and 6. Relapse- can and also do send youths to explore the world of addiction. A peer pressure role-play narrated by Carlos on how he and his friends turned a sixteen year old police officer's son into a 'pothead' explained Prochaska and DiClemente's model working in the opposite direction.

Carlos contends that he was one year younger than Frank, the police officer's son, when this event took place during his tenth grade year. He said he knew that frank knew he and two other friends used marijuana regularly, but "Frank never bothered to join us. I guess because of his dad." He said he and his friends felt uncomfortable, because they felt Frank will 'snitch' on them in a matter of time. Carlos and his friends then decided to pressure Frank to join their dug use habit. They invited Frank to go hang out with them in their favorite alley near the school one afternoon during which time they rolled a marijuana cigarette and offered Frank a puff of the joint. Naturally, Frank refused and told them that his father spends time on the job tracking down people who use drugs. He reminded them that they could go to jail, if they were caught using drugs. Carlos confronted the resistance with the same lecture that got him started two years earlier. He told Frank he was making a stupid mistake by classifying marijuana as a drug. He said marijuana is not a drug because it is not chemically processed like cocaine and the other drugs. He said marijuana is a natural plant and that unlike cocaine marijuana is not addictive. He said his dad smoked marijuana in his school years and got all A's in his classes, including his college classes. He said his dad told him that Frank's dad also used to smoke marijuana when he was in high school…but he cautioned Frank to not ask his dad, because he did not want to get in trouble for gossiping. At that point he turned to his other friend, John, and asked, "What was your grades like in eight grade?" D's and few C's, John intonated. "How long have you been smoking weed now?" Two years, John intonated, again. Carlos then asked John: What are your grades like now? All A's, John said. Take that back, I'm not going to lie, I had two B's last year, John said. Carlos proceeded to educate Frank on some important information on marijuana. He said marijuana was good medicine for cancer, glaucoma, and AIDS. He said almost all the girls in their class smoke marijuana and that is why they (Carlos, John and David) got along so well with the girls. Suddenly, Carlos put a new twist to his lecture. He asserted that in ancient times only wealthy and affluent rulers in Egypt used marijuana. He said one of the Egyptian Pharaohs shared some 'weed' with ancient architects and that is how the Egyptian pyramids were built. Carlos said some Europeans traveled to Egypt during the renaissance and discovered the power of weed. He said those Europeans got too smart for the Queen of England and decided to move to America and start their own country. He said when ordinary citizens found out about the power of weed through one of the early founding fathers daughter, that's when weed became illegal, because "they did not want ordinary citizens to be smart like the rulers." From this point on, the six stages of change were set in motion.

1. Pre-contemplation – Frank told Carlos he did not realize how smart he, Carlos, was. He said Carlos was crazy, though, to think he can convince him to smoke marijuana. "I like the way I am – square." I don't need to change, not even for the girls, he added. Besides, my dad will kill me, if he ever caught me using drugs, Frank said. Yeah! Just like his dad killed him when he was in high school, uh? Carlos quibbled and giggled with his friends.
2. Contemplation – For two days, Carlos and friends deliberately avoided Frank. They hung out at the alley without Frank as they always did. On day three they sent Tiffany to ask Frank why he was not hanging out with his friends any more. Frank met them at the alley on the third day to explain that he was not avoiding them. "Just because I said I was not going to smoke weed the other day does not mean I will never try it. I

do not turn my back on friends just because we do not agree on certain things. Maybe I am just being a daddy's boy." Yeah! Daddy's freaking boy, you're making me feel freaking weird hanging out with the dogs and not being part of the pack, Carlos said. You're probably a snitch; let's get out of here, dogs, Carlos said. "Wait, I'm not a snitch. I will never snitch on my friend. O.k., I will even smoke a puff just to prove it to you." Prove it to us when you buy your own stuff Carlos teased and walked away with his friends.

3. Preparation – Frank saw Carlos in school the next day and apologized for being a butt hole. He said he realized he was being hard on his friends, but they should not expect him to change just like that. That's your problem, Carlos said. "Meet us at the alley after school, that is, if you are not going to snitch on us." Carlos then left and informed the rest of the pack that Frank was in.

4. Action – The boys met after school at the alley. Carlos immediately rolled a joint and said: Frank has something to tell you guys. "I know I have been mean (admit) to you guys, Frank said. I am your friend and friends do not turn their back on each other (commit). I need to stop being a butt hole (abstinence), so pass me the freaking the joint, Dave." You are messing up the rotation, Frank joked. Frank sucked in a lung full of marijuana smoke, paused for a split second and exploded with a thunderous cough. That's my freaking boy! Carlos yelled.

5. Maintenance – I have not given you guys hell for almost three months now, Frank said one day while the boys were hanging out in the alley. Frank was fully initiated into the world of marijuana smoking. He had traded every value his parent taught him regarding drug use. His behavior was changing fast, and so was his desire to use marijuana regularly. About six months after his marijuana-smoking ordeal began, the hard values imbibed in him resurfaced. Frank decided he has had enough. He made a decision to quit using drugs.

6. Relapse – Thirty-six hours after Frank made a decision he was through with marijuana smoking, he found himself at the alley

smoking again. Oops! Relapse had ensued. He realized it
was not going to be easy to just walk away from his new habit.

Carlos admitted Frank was one of few youths whom he had peer-
pressured to use drugs during his days of active drug use. He said
about ninety percent of youths would use drugs from mere strong
suggestion from their favorite peer group. He said boys were very
easily swayed to use drugs if the pressure came from a girl. Consider
a world where one out of every five high school kid use marijuana
regularly, and that one is bent on recruiting more users. This is the
plight of your well behaved, value-ridden, child in public schools
today. Unfortunately, some adults in our society believe marijuana is
not as harmful as experts have tried to convey to the public.

SOCIO-CULTURAL ADDICTION

While genetics may play a key role in addiction, environmental
factors appear to have a strong influence in adolescent and youth drug
use/abuse. Sociocultural factors are strongly linked to all addiction
among youths. Young people tend to seek approval through group
conformity (e.g., accepting the attitudes and practicing the behavior of
friends). Adolescents' views on drug use tend to be molded by the
specific norms of their particular social group. Alcohol/tobacco usage
by close friends is the dominant variable that distinguishes users from
nonusers. Other factors, including rebellion, need for affiliation and
achievement, and cognitive beliefs, are also positively correlated with
the initial onset of alcohol and tobacco use. However, they are not as
influential as peer usage (McCarthy, 1981; Barton, Chassin, Presson
et al, 1982; Chassin Presson, Sherman et al, 1981). In a 12-year
longitudinal investigation of birth cohorts, 1,577 men were studied at
the ages of 19 and 31 (Sieber and Angst, 1989). Questions
concerning their personalities, social backgrounds, and substance use
histories were initially asked. Their responses to these inquiries were
recorded and compared to their self-reports of alcohol, tobacco, and
cannabis use recorded 12 years later. While earlier personality and
social factors were only weakly associated with later alcohol, tobacco,

31

or cannabis usage, substance intake at age 19 was shown to be most accurate indicator of alcohol, tobacco, or cannabis use at age 31.

The behavioral/environmental model states that brain hormones can also be altered by environmental and developmental factors, including chronic physical/emotional stress, peer pressure, media influence and other stimuli, which can motivate people to seek and maintain drug usage. From this perspective, usage is viewed as occurring in graduated levels (Christen and Christen, 1990): Experimental (curiosity seeking and responding to peer pressure); Social/Recreational (sporadic drug seeking on special social occasions); Habitual (patterned usage, involving loss of personal control, but resulting in negligible ill-effects); Abusive (continued usage, in spite of harmful consequences, i.e., uninterrupted smoking patterns displayed by a person with chronic bronchitis); Addictive (abusive use which has become compulsive; i.e., spending increasing amount of time acquiring and using the drug, and focusing in on its effects; seeking to achieve the drug "high" regardless of the consequences, and returning to usage, when attempting to quit without professional help).

Youths are more prone to developing socio-cultural addiction because between adolescence and young adulthood is a period marked by varied growth needs. Erik H. Erikson (1963) in his nine stages of human development asserts the adolescence period is characterized by identity vs. role confusion, while young adulthood is characterized by intimacy vs. isolation. Erikson sees adolescence as consisting of integrating and consolidating psychological growth from earlier stages; finding a sense of personal identity; accepting self as an independent sexual being with personalized needs and desires; developing a sense of self in relationship to immediate others and the world at large; and adopting a personal value system. He describes adulthood as a period for making decisions about life style and career; assuming adult responsibilities; establishing intimate relationships with others; developing adult relationships with family of orientation members.

Socio-cultural addiction centers on the unique rituals surrounding drug use. There is a very socially perceived intimacy that develops during the process. Adolescents who are still struggling with developing a sense of self in relationship to immediate others and the world at large, and young adults who have a weak relationship with family of orientation become particularly vulnerable to socio-cultural addiction. Youths describe in details the social bond that develops when they get together to roll a 'blunt' (marijuana rolled in cigar wrapping). Those oriented from the old school describe sitting around the kitchen table cutting up stashes of marijuana buds, deseeding and picking out hard stems before rolling a 'joint' (marijuana cigarette). Many youths describe the experience as fostering social intimacy. Others spend a great deal of time rolling the joint in stylistic ways. Some are shaped like cones, called 'splits,' and others are rolled fat in the middle, but tapered on each end. Handling the joint itself is ritualistic. Some clutch it between the middle and index fingers, while others hold it between the thumb and index finger. Yet other sophisticated smokers prefer to use an instrument called 'roach clip' to hold the joint.

Daniel Horn, Ph.D., former Director of the National Clearinghouse for smoking and Health, Public Health Services, developed the smoker's (Horn) Self Test, using Tomkins' Model. Horn contends that sensorimotor manipulation during smoking is the main objective of 10 percent of smokers. He says a great deal of enjoyment comes from ritualistically lighting and holding it, flicking the ashes, and watching the smoke curl during exhalation (Horn and Waingrow, 1966; Tomkins, 1968). Some youths are intrigued when new recruits inhale the marijuana smoke and burst out in chronic choke of lung-piercing cough. During these smoking rituals, youths are misinformed about the dangers of smoking. They are told that marijuana is harmless and that it is an all-natural product. One youth said he learned that back in history, only wise rulers smoked marijuana for wisdom. He said when ordinary people discovered the ancient secret, the government decided to make it illegal in other to stop the masses from sharing wisdom. Another youth said smoking marijuana enhanced artistic creativity. Socio-cultural addiction is very powerful in fostering drug abuse HABIT – Highly Automatic Behavior Intensively learned and practiced over a period of Time. Youths often relapse, following a period of abstinence, if they go back to the old socio-cultural milieu. The environment triggers a euphoric recall and relapse usually ensues. The socio-economic environment of a youth is one major indicator of the probability of the percentage of a youth's likelihood to be subjected to negative peer pressure.

Obviously youths who are raised in economically depressed inner cities and low-income neighborhood tend to be subjected to negative role models – parents or significant adults who themselves use drugs and alcohol to cope with social pressures that mark the inequities of a capitalistic society. These youths observe adults from early childhood use drugs and alcohol as social clutches. They see drug and alcohol use as the norm, rather than the exception. In time they too begin to use these substances to cope, just like their adult role models. Do not sigh a gasp of relief, if your child lives in a rural or suburban community. In recent years, drug dealer have found it safer operating in rural areas, since the inner city police have stepped up drug enforcement. A 2002 Monitoring the Future Study (MTF) conducted annually in our nations' schools since 1975 by the University of Michigan through grant from National Institute on Drug Abuse indicates a growing trend in drug use among rural population. "Rural populations serve not only as consumers, but also as traffickers and distributors of these products," wrote Zili Sloboda in his cover story of the December 2002 Counselor Magazine. Sloboda contends that the analysis of the MTF data showed that 8th graders living in rural areas had significantly higher rates of illicit drug use than those living in urban areas. According to the article, past year rates for rural 10th graders also were higher than those for urban 10th graders for all drugs…and, finally, past year rates for rural 12th graders exceeded those of urban seniors for cocaine, crack, amphetamines, inhalants, alcohol, cigarettes, and smokeless tobacco. The article noted: "information from 2001 MTF shows similar results for 8th and 10th graders. In all cases drug use has increased with continuous increases noted for seniors and 10th graders in smaller urban and rural areas." Marijuana use among youths has reaches epidemic proportion. The level of tetrahydrocannabinol (THC), the psychoactive, chemical in marijuana continues to increase as a result of genetic re-engineering, yet, society and policy makers undermine the full impact of marijuana abuse among our youths. The resultant effect is a serious impairment of our marijuana smoking youths in their educational, social, economic, and overall wellbeing.

CHAPTER THREE

DENIAL:
STUMBLING BLOCK IN YOUTH ADDICTION
TREATMENT

Denial is documented in mental health literatures as a natural reaction to external or internal stimulus that threatens a person's physical, mental or emotional equilibrium. The denial process allows a person to minimize, discount or disregard problems that challenge the person's status quo. Many adults go to substance abuse treatment because at some point in time denial mechanisms tend to break down due to compelling evidence to the contrary. The compelling reasons may be, but are not limited to, loss of jobs, family, membership to social circle, degrading public arrests by police officers, to mention but a few. For most youths, marijuana use provides the much needed social identity that most adolescents and youths crave. Other youths perceive themselves as invulnerable, thereby exacerbating the denial process. When it comes to youth substance use/abuse treatment, they are almost always forced into treatment by their parents, youth authority, courts, or some institution of learning or skill training. The corresponding resistance to treatment by the youth increases the denial propensity, which in turn, empowers addiction and allows it to exert ultimate control. In time, the youth loses touch of his/her reality base or blatantly chose to ignore reality.

Denial is one of several ultimately unconscious, self-protective defense mechanisms that youths use to justify marijuana use. Over a long period of time using marijuana, these under-listed defense mechanisms become reality:

- Denial: the belief or insistence that a source of distress is non-existence; e.g., smoking marijuana has nothing to do with me dropping out of high school. In fact, I used to make straight 'A's in 9th grade smoking weed. Besides, it's not like I am addicted to weed. I can stop when I want to.

- Suppression: conscious exclusion of painful desires or thoughts from awareness; e.g., a youth who smokes marijuana daily may say to a counselor during intake assessment: "I am not addicted. I don't smoke every day. I quit for a whole year before" (he actually quit for two weeks at an attempt to get a job).
- Rationalization: the presentation of a socially acceptable, yet inaccurate, reason to justify a questionable behavior; e.g., "my dad is an alcoholic. He stresses me out when he gets drunk, so I smoke weed to relax."
- Displacement: the masking of actual goals or motives by substituting more acceptable ones in their place; e.g., I don't spend my money on weed. I only smoke it when my friends offer it to me (he is around his friends several times a day, smoking marijuana).
- Projection: the disguising of one's own problematic behaviors by ascribing them to another; e.g., "my mom has been smoking crack for as long as I can remember. My dad is an alcoholic. Everybody in my family is messed up."
- Sublimation: the discharge of physical tension or stress by excessively engaging in socially acceptable behavior; e.g., an alcoholic youth who says to his counselor: "I take a few drinks to relax. It's not like I'm doing drugs."
- Intellectualization: the removal of feeling content from a stressful situation or the exclusive use of cognition in response to events which would normally produce anxiety; e.g., a youth tells his counselor that most successful people he knows smoke marijuana. "I rap better when I'm high. Even former, President Bill, Clinton used to smoke weed."

Many youths live in denial of marijuana use for various reasons: 1. Some have established no reality base. These youths usually may have been raised in an atmosphere of denial and chaotic living, where they had no opportunity to learn healthy, functional responses from positive, parental role models. 2. Some youths may have lost touch with reality. This may be due to short/long term memory impairment caused by excessive physical/emotional stress and chemical usage or the drug-related loss of 'here and now' living experiences. 3. Other youths chose to distort or ignore reality. This group is mostly controlled by their marijuana addiction. They tend to distort reality by rationalizing away personal responsibility and ignoring both their limits and the consequences of their behaviors. As denial continues to build up and intensify these youths begin to formulate coping mechanisms that allow them to en-cyst themselves from the internal or external stimulus that creates the reality they seek to escape. Finally, these youths begin to engage in self-defeating behavior as they move further away from reality.

SELF-DEFEATING BEHAVIOR (SDB) SYNDROME

The mid 1960s was marked by a social upheaval. The Flower Children or the so-called Hippies radically embarked upon a mission to rejuvenate the existing social other through self-expression. The Flower Children purportedly hoped to achieve a new world order through peace, love and happiness. By 1967, this movement had gathered momentum. Many young people headed to San Francisco in search of the illusive new social order, propelled by a state of mind that was driven by the genius of two major psychoactive substances, marijuana and lysergic acid diethylamide (LSD). Later in that decade amphetamine and its derivative, methamphetamine, were introduced as part of the catalyst to fuel the new social other. As the ingenious minds that envisioned a new social order began to be warped by methamphetamine, a massive campaign was launched against it; "Speed kills." In the aftermath, those who overindulged in the use of LSD profoundly stymied their brainpower to stupor. Most, literally, fried their brains. Indeed, the very essence they thought would revolutionize the world now worked against them. This exemplifies the classic self-defeating behavior (SDB).

Robert Ackerman, (June 17, 2002) defines SDB as cognitive behavioral model in which an action or attitude that once helped an individual cope with an adverse situation later turned against that individual. SDB emanates from self-defeating thought processes. The more an individual practice SDB, the more the individual makes adjustment to self-defeating thought processes. This syndrome is sometimes described as 'stinking thinking' in substance abuse therapeutic communities. Over a period of time, SDB becomes relegated into the subconscious. There are four characteristics associated with SDB: 1. SDB helps an individual deal with an adverse or unfavorable situation, 2. The behavior is almost always based on a faulty belief system, which, in turns guarantees a faulty conclusion, 3. It may not have been the best course of action at the time, but it helped deal with the emotional pain associated with an adverse or unfavorable situation, and finally, 4. SDB guarantees the consequence the individual tried to avoid in the first place.

SDB has always been a subject of interest to psychologists and clinicians. Sigmund Freud spoke of the 'success neurosis' consisting of four motives: a need to achieve, a fear of success, a fear of failure, and a desire to fail. The fear of failure can cause a person to be nervous (and not do well) or to give up; however, it can also cause a person to work very hard, just like the need to achieve. While working with youths at Job Corps, it is not uncommon to see youths who are making immense progress in their vocational pursuit suddenly mess up or drop out. Cudney (1981) in his book, *Man Against Himself*, suggests that SDB is caused by our reluctance to face reality. By failing (while pretending to be trying to succeed) we deny our responsibility for what is happening. That way, our goof-ups can continue but "they aren't my fault." Most youths who are forced to go to Job Corps tend to resent the idea, which may cause them to want to fail. Failure can serve a useful purpose to such a youths: get sympathy, frustrate or disappoint his/her parent(s), and/or confirm the belief that he/she is not ready for the program. Although SDB can be anything – laziness, poor habits, drug use, alcoholism, anger, or jealousy, marijuana use is a more common type of SDB among youths. Once the marijuana use becomes a habit and productivity begins to dwindle (a predictable sine qua non), many youths turn to SDB to justify their behavior or seemingly maintain their perceived status quo. Consistent with Gilmer's (1975) signs of inferiority many youths who engage in marijuana use/abuse usually exhibit the following symptoms: over-reaction to criticism, tendency to feel criticized, avoidance of others, an excessively positive response to flattery, inability to lose graciously, and urges to put down others. When a youth begins to show the above listed signs, usually something is going on in his/her life.

Most self-defeating behavior begin as childhood experience carried over into youth and sometimes adulthood. In chapter one we read about Ashley's resentment toward her stepfather. Many youths who use marijuana as a coping mechanism have very similar stories of childhood experiences that later led to addiction to marijuana. A child is super-sensitive to feelings and can even be sensitive to other's thoughts. There is no way of making comparisons or having a perspective on things other than what is happening at that moment. The moment is what is real. The moment is what is eternal. To a child what is experienced now, is irrefutable fact. The child's mind and senses take in everything literally and with total acceptance. Since children experience everything as revolving around them, they are apt to blame themselves for anything that is upsetting. Children do not experience reality outside of themselves. They are the center of the world. All revolves around them. Because of this, children tend to assume that they are responsible for everything that happens. They have no other perspective to understand anything else. As a result, children often view conflict as being purposefully directed towards them. Imagine what it feels like to interpret stressful experiences as meaning you are not worthy, lovable, safe, or good, that you are guilty, or that your feelings and needs are unimportant. This is the meaning children often give to their experience. Fortunately, parents and other significant adults in a child's life are constantly reassuring a child with love, safety, feeling of worthiness, and removing the feeling of guilt from the child. Unfortunately, as society unfold and undergo social metamorphosis, sometimes these vital roles of parent and significant adults diminish. As the divorce rate increases, the number of single parent family increases and significant adults are more and more becoming a thing of the past; children are faced with a new plight with uncertain future. In the midst of balancing two jobs, bills and family, childcare sometimes takes the back burner position. A glimpse at the daily news reveals countless instances of children being forgotten in cars and left to suffocate; children being molested by what used to be significant adults in the children's lives; children being flooded into underprivileged foster homes due to parental neglect; children killing their peers or parents, ad infinitum.

A child, like any living being, needs to feel worthy, loved, valued, and safe. If these essential emotional needs are threatened, it becomes a survival issue. A child, who does not feel worthy, loved, valued, and safe intuitively senses the life threatening possibility of abandonment. Even a hint of threat alerts the child. The stronger the threat is perceived, the greater the necessity of adopting defenses to survive. Not feeling loved or valued is a survival issue for a child. In order to understand our defenses, we must understand this. A child who is verbally or physically attacked, emotionally or physically abandoned, neglected, ignored, or lied to, does not have the capacity to defend himself or find another home. The child will do whatever he can to survive where he is. He does not have the perspective that things may change. His moment is experienced as an eternity. He will respond in the only way he can in order to cope. When you see through the eyes of a child, all responses are appropriate. When childhood defenses are carried forward into youth life, they are usually inappropriate and self-defeating. Most of our defenses have been carried forward from childhood into the present. Though the reason for the defense may be outmoded and long forgotten, the reaction still persists. The defense becomes an unconscious habit (Hill, 2002).

A child is, indeed, a helpless victim of circumstances and of the behaviors and attitude of those who raise him. A child needs to have a sense of autonomy and personal power. If he doesn't have a sense of having a say with others he learns to feel like a victim. He learns that others cannot be trusted and do not care about helping him fill his needs. This may cause feelings of self-pity and helplessness. These feelings get carried forward in time and grow to be major self-defeating response. Many youths join gangs because they feel the gang members will help them fill their needs and offer them care. Others fulfill their need for belongingness by joining gangs. In turn, by becoming members of gangs self-pity disappears and helplessness is replaces with survival instincts. Eventually, the very coping mechanisms that allow these youths resolve feelings of ambivalence, hopelessness, helplessness and victim status will guarantee that they get exactly the same feelings and emotions they were trying to escape in the first place. For such is the very nature of self-defeating behavior. Many adults, like these youths, are unconsciously caught in their past, unaware that they are responding to a forgotten memory and acting out a no longer appropriate response in the present. The ego needs to rationalize behavior so it finds a way to justify the response. Many adult alcoholics have said, "If you were married to my wife, you'll drink too." Or this is just the way I am. I was born with this temperament. I inherited it from my parents." In truth, these defenses were created from childhood decisions. In fact, this all shows the human innate ability to survive physically, emotionally, and spiritually. It is a testimony of our ability to learn, says Hill.

TERMINAL UNIQUENESS SYNDROME

Less than 40 percent of seized marijuana was grown in the U.S. fifteen to thirty years ago. Colombia and Mexico were the sources of most marijuana. The marijuana of that era contained less than five percent of delta-9-tetrahydrocannabinol, THC (the psychoactive ingredient in marijuana). Little mention was made about the medical aspects of marijuana, except those who smoked the so-called loco weed from Mexico were thought to be crazy. Today, more than 60 percent of seized marijuana is currently grown and cultivated predominantly in northern California and Pacific Northwest, particularly British Columbia. In 2000, U.S. and Canadian Customs seized more than 4,000 pounds of highly potent marijuana grown in British Columbia. Majority of the marijuana is grown hydroponically (without soil) under powerful 1000-watt halide lamps with ventilation and exhaust systems to reduce the heat from the lamps and the smell from the vegetation. Hydroponically grown marijuana, such as the 'B.C. (British Columbia) bud' now contains more than 12 percent THC. By contrast, the average potency of Mexican or common domestic marijuana was about three percent, and that of Colombian grown 'Sinsemilla' was 4.6 percent. Hybrid, genetically re-engineered, marijuana seeds are now easily purchased online through the internet or from High Times and other sub-culture magazines for as little as 10 seed for 80 cent to $1.50 per seed, depending on potency. Many adults, especially those who were youths during the sixties, tend to view marijuana as not harmful or less harmful than other drugs, we cannot discount the dangers of the genetically re-engineered brands of marijuana as new research and findings become available. David S. Brinks, a colleague at the St. Louis University School of Medicine presented a recent case analysis to the Society for Pediatric Pathology. Three teenage boys ages 15-17 who sought medical treatment for headache, ataxia and lethargy after using marijuana became comatose and two died within a week of seeking treatment. All three tested positive for no other drugs than marijuana. Brinks noted that toxic effect of a contaminant of the marijuana might have caused the stroke that killed the teenage boys. Aside from genetically increasing the level of THC in the average marijuana sold on the streets today, many youths say that most of the marijuana they use in recent times are adulterated with one or more of club drugs such as ecstasy, rohypnol, ketamine, gamma-hydroxybutyrate (GHB) or methamphetamine. These contaminants increase the risk of severe health problems.

Marijuana is the most widely used illicit drug among today's youth. According to the National Household Survey on Drug Abuse (2001), among kids age 12-17 who use drugs, approximately 60 percent use marijuana only. Moreover, the number of 8th graders who have used the drug has doubled in the last decade from 10.2 percent in 1991 to 20.4 percent in 2001, (Monitoring the future, 2001). Contrary to popular belief, research has now established that marijuana is addictive. In fact, more kids enter treatment each year for marijuana than for all other illicit drugs combined. About sixty percent of teens currently in drug treatment have a primary marijuana diagnosis. We noted in the preceding paragraph that marijuana is more potent and its effects can be more intense today than ever before. Unfortunately, some significant adults in our community are sending mixed messages to our children through advocacy for the so-called medical marijuana use. Any physician that has good training and ethical standing of any type can attest that smoke-able medical marijuana is an antithesis. In medicine, it is not common practice to destroy one organ, the lung, so as to save the eye from glaucoma. Beside, marinol (a synthetic THC and a more effective alternative to smoke-able marijuana) has been proven to be a more efficient medicine than marijuana in treating cancer patients and other in that class. Yet states like California and Arizona, including 22 others have passed legislations that attempt to authorize medical use of marijuana. Indeed, proponents of medical marijuana use are shamefully trying to con voters through deceptive ballot referenda exploiting the ill and dying. Keith Stroup, founder of the National Organization for the Reform of Marijuana Law or NORML told Emory University audience in 1979 that medical marijuana would be used as a red herring to give marijuana a good name. By the same token, Richard Cowan, writing for the pro-drug High Times Magazine, described the medical model as spearheading a strategy for the legalization of marijuana in 1997. Despite flimsy arguments about the medical benefits of smoke-able marijuana, the truth remains that marijuana, especially the hybrids of today, is a dangerous drug that destroys the user subtly.

Unlike cigarette smoke, marijuana smoke contains more tar and carbon monoxide, which facilitates deposition of carbon particles in the alveoli inside the lungs. Regular marijuana users often develop breathing problems including chronic coughing and wheezing. Asthma is a common childhood disease. Smoking marijuana makes any ailing condition like asthma worse. Smoking marijuana leads to changes in the brain that are like those caused by cocaine, heroin and alcohol. In fact, because marijuana is fat soluble, it deposits in brain fat tissue cells and becomes neurotoxin over a long period of time using it. Boys who use marijuana tend to develop unusually large breast and experience decrease in testosterone count. Girls, who use marijuana experience disrupted menstrual cycle, develop deep voice due to increase in testosterone and grow facial hair. The immune systems of marijuana smokers are generally weak, thereby subjecting them to frequent battles with common ailments. According to the National Household Survey on Drug Abuse, adolescents age 12 to 17 who use marijuana weekly are nine times more likely than non-users to experiment with illegal drugs or alcohol, five times more likely to steal and nearly four times more like to engage in violence. For young users, marijuana can lead to increased anxiety, panic attacks, depression and other mental health problems. One study found that adolescents associated social withdrawal, anxiety and depression, attention problems and thought of suicide with past-year marijuana use. Some common side effects and physical effects include memory, sleepiness, paranoia, altered time perception, amotivational syndrome, tremors, nausea, headache, reduced blood flow to the brain and breathing problems.

A long-term study published in the June 2002 issue of the Journal of Adolescent Health linked adolescent drug use with health problem in early adulthood. Subjects in their mid to late twenties who had used drugs as teens reported more health problems than those who had never used drugs. Health problems included: increased incidence of respiratory conditions, such as colds and sinus infections; cognitive problems, such as difficulty in concentrating, remembering, and learning; and headaches, dizziness, and vision problems. The NIDA-funded study also found that rebelliousness, distrust of authority, and risk-taking behavior in early adolescence and peer influences in middle adolescence were precursors to later drug use, which, in turn, led to increased health problems. These findings are from a 22-year study that tracked the self-reported substance abuse and health histories of more than 600 youths through their early and mid teen years into early adulthood. Scientists from the Mount Sinai School of Medicine and Columbia University started collecting data on the children in 1975, when the subjects were one through 10 years of age. Four follow-up interviews were conducted in 1983, 1986, 1992, and 1997. By the time of the last interview, the average subject was 27 years old. Lead investigator Dr. Judith S. Brooks published the study in June 2002.

One of the most debilitating aspects of marijuana use is the socio-psychological transformation that youths undergo when they become very indulgent in the marijuana habit. Physiologically and pharmacologically, marijuana is an addictive drug, although most youths do not know that. Over a long period of usage, many youths sustain cognitive problems that sink them deeper into self-defeating behavior, which further creates undue challenges to treatment. Social psychologists have discovered that one of the most powerful determinants of human behavior stems from our need to preserve a stable, positive self-concept; that is, to maintain a relative favorable view of ourselves, particularly when we encounter evidence that contradicts our typically rosy self-image (Wicklund and Brehm, 1998). We pretty much want to see ourselves as reasonable, moral and smart. When we are confronted with information implying we may have behaved in ways that are irrational, immoral, or stupid, we will experience discomfort. This feeling of discomfort is what social psychologists call cognitive dissonance. Leon Festinger (1957) was first to investigate the precise workings of this powerful phenomenon. Dissonance theory asserts that people feel most dissonance and upset when they behave in ways that threaten their self-image. This is upsetting because it forces people to confront the discrepancy between who they think they are and how they have behaved. Generally speaking, cognitive dissonance occurs when we do something that tends to make us feel absurd, stupid, or immoral – as defined by our own standards of reasonableness, intelligence, and morality.

There are three basic ways to reduce dissonance when it occurs: 1. Change the behavior to bring it in line with the dissonant cognition; for example, a youth is caught smoking marijuana in his room by his parents. His parents express their disappointment in the youth's behavior and legal/moral implications of smoking marijuana. The youth may reduce dissonance by deciding not to ever use marijuana again. 2. Justify the behavior through changing one of the dissonant cognition; for example, the youth from our preceding example may elect to not ever smoke in the house again and thereby, reducing the dissonance associated with getting caught by his parents. Or 3. Justify the behavior by adding new cognitions. When people are faced with situations in which they have little control of or have lost control of, they tend to add new cognitions. Rick Gibbons and his colleagues (1997) found that heavy smokers who attend a smoking cessation clinic, quit smoking for a while and then relapsed into heavy smoking again, actually succeeded in lowering their perception of the dangers of smoking. These smokers become very creative in justifying their smoking; for example, some might try to convince themselves that data linking cigarette smoking to cancer are inconclusive. Others will try to add new cognitions – for example, the erroneous belief that filters trap most of the harmful chemicals and thus reduce the threat of cancer. Some will add a cognition that allows them to focus on the vivid exception: "Look at uncle Willie – he's 92 years old and he has been smoking a pack a day since he was 12. That proves it's not always bad for you." Marijuana smoking youths usually add new cognitions by rationalization or over-justification that is often based on false premise, sometimes referred to as "Stinking Thinking."

Ed's Story

One of the brilliant youths from Job Corps, Ed, landed himself in a rationalization trap (the potential for dissonance reduction to produce a succession of self-justifications that ultimately result in a chain of stupid or immoral actions), which eventually took his life. Ed was the classic case of egomorphism: the tendency to attribute one's own need, desire, motives, etc, to others, sometimes referred to as projection. Ed has learned to reduce dissonance by attributing his flaws to his parents. He claimed his mother was an alcoholic right from the time of his birth. He said his father gave him a puff of marijuana when he was five years old; therefore, it was not his fault that he is an alcoholic and a "weed head" (someone addicted to marijuana). At age 19, Ed had developed strong ego strength and had become comfortable in his ego syntonism. He proudly tells the story of his father, whose only mistake was crossing the line from marijuana smoking to using crack cocaine and finally ending up in jail for murder. Dissonance-reducing behavior is ego-defensive behavior. It can be useful because it keeps our egos from being continually battered; it provides us with a feeling of stability and high self-esteem. Dissonance-reducing behavior can be dangerous as well. The tendency to justify our past behavior can lead us into an escalation of rationalizations that can be disastrous. Ed said his father had taught him street survival skills. He bragged about being able to survive with little or nothing, if left in the middle of the dessert. He said by the time he was 12 years old; he was smoking marijuana on a regular basis. He said he was also selling drugs and had a pocket full of money, while in middle school. He said he was a straight 'A' student. He attributed his good grade to smoking marijuana – a story that is highly questionable, since he did not finish high school. He said his father was a smart hard-working man, who provided for his family, until he started smoking crack cocaine.

Ed said he was smarter than his father, because he will NEVER use any other drugs, besides the "God given, all-natural," marijuana. Ed's rationalization allowed him to reduce dissonance associated with the fact that at age 19 he was a high school drop out, whose father was serving 25 to life sentence for murder due to the same very behavior that he (Ed) was promoting. He said most of his creative ideas come from smoking marijuana. Ed's mother was an alcoholic. She had turned to prostitution shortly after Ed's father was incarcerated. Ed hated his mother for her behavior. He often said that if his mother will just leave the booze alone and smoke weed, she would be o.k. However, he fails to acknowledge that he, too, was an alcoholic. He often said that he could stop drinking if he wanted. Asked why he wouldn't, he often said there was nothing wrong with a having a few beers, as long as it was not abused. He said he enjoys drinking after smoking marijuana to quench the thirst associated with smoking marijuana. He said he knows when to stop, unlike his mother who does not know her limits. After a few weeks of hard-core disposition in group therapy, Ed finally got in touch with his feelings in group one afternoon and cried. Once again, dissonance set in. Ed caught himself, laughed sarcastically, and said he was just faking a cry, because he knew the author expected him to do just that.

Once self-justification, rationalization, and extreme dissonance-reducing behavior sets in among youths who use marijuana or any other drugs, they feel terminally unique. This terminal uniqueness syndrome exacerbates drug abuse and will usually land youths in Youth Authority, Juvenile Hall, jail or even death. Such was the plight of Ed. He had been to Juvenile Hall for troubled youths in California, spent time in foster homes and Youth Authority before emancipating to the Job Corps training program. Ironically, he had skills and potentials to become a good welder, his chosen vocational skill training. Within four months of stay at the Job Corps program, he had completed and attained his GED (high school equivalent). He was doing very well in the welding program. During this time, he had managed to abstain from using marijuana for about ninety days, although he drank moderately during the weekends. He visited his girlfriend one weekend and decided he was not coming back to Job Corps. Evidently, he had gone back to his familiar drug use environment, experienced euphoric recall and relapsed. He was on AWOL status for about nine days. Finally, he called the author and stated that he was not coming back to Job Corps. He said he needed to stay home and take care of his girlfriend. All attempts to get him to return to the program proved futile. Three months after Ed left the Job Corps program, he made the front page of the local section of the newspaper. He died in a car accident. Autopsy revealed his blood alcohol level was three times the legal limit. Ed's story is the norm, rather than the exception in working with many youths. Somehow, one of the dangerous side effects of marijuana smoking as a self-defeating behavior is the terminal uniqueness syndrome.

Youths who engage in marijuana abuse feel a sense of uniqueness. Many youths have asserted in treatment group that their special circumstance that justifies using marijuana is different from those of their peers. Oftentimes, they feel invulnerable. Other times they get a false illusion that smoking marijuana enhances performance of certain skills. One youth said he raps better after smoking a blunt (marijuana wrapped in cigar leaf). Successful members of his therapy group challenged his illusion. He claimed he had recorded tapes at home to prove his point. His group members asked him to bring the tapes back to group over the weekend. He did. We all had a laugh, including him, after we heard the tapes sober. Part of the terminal uniqueness is "hip, slick and cool" disposition. Youths who smoke marijuana consider themselves uniquely qualified to take on the world. They walk with a stylistic gait, dress roughly flamboyant and talk with special drug culture slang. This particular disposition is what many a youth in middle and high school find attractive. It becomes a powerful element in recruiting prospective marijuana smokers. Adolescents and youth struggle with identity crisis as it is. To be presented with an identity that, from all outward appearances, seems sophisticated is a final assault on reasoning. Many youths will do just about anything to be part of the hip, slick, and cool crowd. Those who join the local gang do so mostly because of the hip slick and cool attraction of the gang members, coupled with the promise of protection, care and unconditional love (or so they say) that members offer their prospective recruits.

Many youths who use marijuana see themselves as bodily and mentally different from others. They feel on top of their games and over a considerable period of time, their illusion, denial and dissonance-reducing behavior become their reality. One youth, James, tested positive (1,020 nanograms of THC per millimeter of blood) for marijuana on entry into the Job Corps program. He denied he had ever used marijuana before. He claimed that nobody in his family ever used drugs. Forty-five days after his entry, during his follow-up drug test, he stated this was the second time he tested positive for drugs due to administrative error. He said he was discharged from the Navy the first time around because of positive drug test. He said 'they' later found out that the sergeant who tested him had used the urine collection cup they gave him for the urinalysis as ashtray for his marijuana cigarette. Three months into therapy James admitted he is a marijuana addict and that everyone in his family used drugs for as long as he can remember. There are many youths out there who fit in Ed and James' description - Youths who have become impaired from smoking marijuana. For all those youths, there is a solution. Marijuana addiction is treatable, but early intervention is important in the treatment process.

CHAPTER FOUR

BUILDING THERAPEUTIC ALLIANCE

There are many substance abuse treatment facilities nationwide. However, there are only very few exclusively devoted to youths and adolescents. When youths are put in the treatment programs with adults, it creates a special challenge, and oftentimes, it creates a chaotic atmosphere that disrupts the whole treatment process. This is because youths see adults as role models and seeing them in treatment depicts an image of failure on the part of adults. This, in turn, leads to disrespect for adults in treatment, which affects the smooth functioning of treatment groups. On the other hand, adults tend to look at youths as being too young to indulge in substance use. They see these youths as renegades who defied their parents' advises, so naturally adults in treatment look at youths in treatment with disdain. Once again, there is conflict of expectation, which leads to friction in group. Working with youths in treatment poses a special challenge. Often youths go to treatment because they are forced to, not because they come to the realization that marijuana use has direct correlation with their setback or special social/vocational circumstance. Further, many youths lose faith in their parents and other adults long before getting to treatment. On arrival to treatment, they are faced with the same adults with whom they already "have problems with," coupled with the fact that these youths already suffer from terminal uniqueness, which means that adults will not understand their plights, anyway.

In chapter six we will examine and encourage the use of different therapeutic approaches in working with youths, but generally, behavioral, cognitive-behavioral and group therapies are the most widely used methods. Behavioral therapy, or behavioral modification, is a psychological technique based on the premise that specific, observable, maladaptive, badly adjusted, or self-defeating behaviors, can be modified by learning new, more appropriate behaviors. Behavioral therapy can be a useful treatment tool in an array of mental illnesses and symptoms of mental illness that involve maladaptive behavior, such as substance abuse, aggressive behavior, anger management, and anxiety disorders. Cognitive-behavioral therapy is an action-oriented form of psychosocial therapy that assumes that maladaptive, or faulty, thinking patterns cause maladaptive behavior and negative emotions. Maladaptive behavior refers to behavior that is counter-productive or interferes with everyday living. Treatment focuses on changing an individual's thoughts in order to change his or her behavior and emotional state. Theoretically, cognitive-behavioral therapy can be employed in any situation in which there is a pattern of unwanted behavior accompanied by distress and impairment. Group therapy is a form of psychosocial treatment where a small group of patients meet regularly to talk, interact, and discuss problems with each other and the group leader (therapist) directs and modifies the flow of interaction. Group therapy attempts to give individuals a safe and comfortable place where they can work out problems and emotional issues. Patients can gain insight into their own thoughts and behavior, and offer suggestions and support to others. In addition, patients who have a difficult time with interpersonal relationships can benefit from the social interactions that are a basic part of the group therapy experience.

One of the most consistently critical factors in the psychotherapy process is the working alliance, commonly called therapeutic alliance, which has come to be seen as a necessary component of counseling, regardless of theoretical framework. In fact, therapeutic alliance has been shown to account for 30 to 50 percent of the variance in outcome measurement across a range of studies (Gelso & Carter, 1985; Horvath & Luborsky, 1993). Unfortunately, many adult counselors do not fully understand the importance of developing an effective therapeutic alliance with youths or they do not have the necessary training to understand its importance. Robert Schwebel (Counselor, February 2002) observes: Nowhere is the deviation from the traditional counseling more obvious than in drug treatment for adolescents, which could best be characterized as a mad rush for abstinence. Youths who enter treatment are barraged with information about the harmfulness of drugs. When they talk about what they like about drugs, treatment professionals generally make counter-arguments or accuse them of glamorizing drugs. Tremendous pressure is brought to bear on young people to get them to say that they will quit "using." He contends that in most cases it is fairly easy to get drug-abusing adolescents to say that they want to be drug-free. "What often happens in drug treatment for adolescents is that young people make an insincere commitment to abstinence," he said. He added that ultimately young people accede by "faking it." This he asserts explains the high rate of relapse, following adolescent treatment.

YOUTHS IN TREATMENT DEMAND 'RESPEKT'

Developing therapeutic alliance with marijuana abusing youths in treatment, school, church, or at home requires unorthodox, yet well formulated technique. Many marijuana abusing youths 'demand respect,' although they have no clue what the word respect means, nor are they able to spell it for the most part. One college drug and alcohol counselor intern (Debbie) in the Job Corps youth treatment program (TEAP) was frustrated when she attempted to establish therapeutic alliance with one of the youths in treatment. The counselor intern had received several weeks of training and was anxious to begin handling her own clients. It was common practice to assign interns with the most challenging youth, based on initial assessment record. That way, the interns were able to learn hands-on as the program director (TEAP Specialist) mediated and guided the treatment process back on track.

Leon's Story
Debbie was assigned to work with a youth named Leon, whose middle name is Andre, who preferred to be called Dre, because he "hated" the name Leon. His father who was in jail was also named Leon. Initial assessment indicates Dre was marijuana dependent, had been in Juvenile Hall several times for various offenses, does not know his father because his father had been in jail since he was three years old. During assessment he blatantly said there was nothing the treatment program can do for him, because he loved smoking blunts (marijuana rolled with cigar paper) and he was not about to stop. He

53

said smoking marijuana gives him inspiration. Debbie told Dre during a joint assessment/treatment planning with the TEAP Specialist that she would address him as Leon, not Dre, because it was important for him to change his street attitude and begin to straighten out his behavior in preparation for the professional world that comes after his vocational skills training. I immediate knew Debbie had lost him. Dre responded: "Who the f--k are you to tell me what I should be called?" The TEAP Specialist quickly intervened: "Chill Dre. Home girl was just tripping. She don't mean none of that what she said." Dre made an attempt to direct the course of the treatment: "Look, tell fat A - - to stay out of this. I just want to talk to you. I don't want her in my mix." The TEAP Specialist had had enough of Dre and immediately regained control of his client and added Debbie on Dre's good book: "Look Dre, I know Debbie 'dissed' (disrespected you) you, but two wrongs don't make a right, so let's shake hands and call it even. Debbie show some respect and call the man his real name." Three months into treatment another client in group offended Dre, because the client called him Dre. He said he did not appreciate being called street names. "I just want to be myself, 'Leon.' You got problem with that?" He asked. It was always fascinating to see the transformation from hard core, street-wise, I'm in control, attitude to civil, respectable and responsible disposition as youths go through successful treatment. However, establishing the initial rapport can be a healthy challenge.

It is important to understand youth culture and buy into that culture, even if momentarily, in other to work with youths successfully. Another college intern, Pete, learned the hard way. Pete was a very bright young man. He himself was in recovery from substance abuse. He decided to take up a career in substance abuse counseling as part of his vocational rehabilitation. He was a construction worker before drug and alcohol abuse took toll on his career. He spent six months in an in-house residential treatment. He was convinced that going back to construction work will trigger a relapse, hence he decided on a new career line. Pete spent five years in the streets, totally wasted on drug abuse. He prides himself as knowing all about addiction. He felt like his personal experience equipped him with more than enough skill to deal with youths in treatment. After all, he usually says: "I've been there, done that." Pete said he started using marijuana in eight grade and continued through high school until after high school when he discovered cocaine and methamphetamine. Pete was about to discover that it takes more than being an ex drug abuser to be an effective counselor. Pete was assigned to work with Nicole.

Nicole's Story

Nicole started using alcohol at the age of twelve. At age thirteen, she began using marijuana and two years after, she became a "twicker" (methamphetamine user). Nicole said she is a devil worshipper. Her father was a Hell's Angels motorcycle rider who was never home. She said her father was a stone alcoholic. She said her mother hated her because she is pretty and her best friends are all guys. Nicole loves to wear black outfits. She wears a military-style black boot, a black pants (cut off right below the knees) worn with a black belt that has metallic chrome studs, a black blouse with low neck to reveal her bosoms, and a black 'Matrix-style' over-coat. Her nails are painted black and she wore a heavy black lipstick. She had about fifteen piercing ranging from two chrome studs in her navel, three on each ear, to one on each eye lid, two on her nose, two on her lips and one on her tongue. She said she had other piercing on other parts of her body. She had a heart-shaped tattoos on her bosom, a skull and bone tattooed to her neck, a death-like creature tattooed on the back of her waist line and the numbers 666 tattooed across each knuckle. During final assessment/treatment planning, Pete told her that her attention-seeking outfit did not intimidate him, because he too had "been there done that." He said it was time to make a change for the better. "Look at me, I used to be hip, slick and cool like you, but now I realize it was all stupidity. I am here to help you change all that. I probably spilt more booze than you ever drank and wasted more dope than you ever used, but today I've got my life straight. I can help you turn around," Pete said. For a split second, I could hear the honesty and sincerity in Pete's voice. His heart was talking, but the job ahead of him required more than heart. Pete had very good intentions, but then, the road to hell was also paved with good intentions. Nicole listened to him in total dismay and disgust. She suddenly yelled: "That was so, so, very wrong of you to judge me. Don't blame me for you being sloppy – spilling your drink and all. You sound just like my father. Oh! I hate you."

It was time to restore order and control, the TEAP Specialist told himself. "Look Pete, Nicole was right. You are judging her by her appearance. I know that deep down she is probably one of the coolest persons you will ever meet. Besides, it cost about $30 for each of those piercing. You got to recognize." Nicole's eyes were wide in amazement, when she realized that the TEAP Specialist knew how much the piercing cost. Almost immediately, an alliance was developing between them. But, that was not all. The TEAP Specialist continued: "I like your boot, Nicole. Did you buy them from France? I saw those same boots in France last summer. I know those jacket got to be real expensive, and I know you got your T-shirt from Britney Spear concert." Nicole spent the next ten minutes talking about Britney Spear and how she is so, so, cool, while we listened and enjoyed rapport building up. "Look Nicole, let's forget about what Pete said earlier and start over. So, what was your first drug of choice…?" Developing therapeutic alliance with young people requires tact and special handling. As adults, we are too quick to judge youths. Ironically, once we develop bias towards youths, they tend to perceive our bias and they reciprocate our bias. We were able to penetrate Nicole's iron clad defense by acknowledging her style and appearance. This is not to say that we encourage her bizarre look, nor do we intend to abet her so-called devil worshipping. The primary purpose during this initial contact is to establish a warm and supportive milieu on which adequate assessment will be developed. Assessment is an ongoing process. However, the initial client assessment is very important in the treatment-planning phase. Failure to establish a good rapport and therapeutic alliance with the youth may lead to faulty or incomplete diagnosis of the youth's problem. This, in turn, would mean faulty or wrong "prescription" of an appropriate treatment. We will discuss assessment further in chapter five.

Assessment can be a very tedious exercise, depending on the size and modality of the treatment facility. Often it may involve a multi-disciplinary team consisting of a substance abuse counselor, a medical doctor, a psychologist/psychiatrist, and a dentist. However, in a social model treatment setting, a substance abuse counselor, school counselor, clergy, or even parent can get the preliminary assessment done. A complete assessment is not likely to be completed in a one-hour session. It is recommended that full assessment with youths be broken down into at least three sessions. The first session is the most important and should not exceed 15 to 20 minutes. Youths generally have short attention span. Besides, most youths come to treatment not by choice. Oftentimes, they have not come to grips with the correlation of their marijuana habit and the consequences associated with the habit. In fact, for most youths, marijuana use is inconsequential. Any attempt to impose upon a youth any suggestion that using marijuana has social or health implication may lead to disagreement by way of debate or outright rebellion in some instances. Once a counselor, clergy, parent or teacher puts her/himself in a position of debate about the consequences of marijuana use, therapeutic alliance is broken; therefore treatment planning becomes stymied or compromised. That not withstanding, many youths arrive to treatment within 48 hours of last drug use. During this time, the blood is still saturated with drugs and psychotic symptoms may interfere with attention span. Mario exemplifies what happens when initial assessment is not limited to 15 to 20 minutes.

After the Nicole experience, Pete shared some intellectual thoughts with the TEAP Specialist. He said he was pleased with his training as an Intern and noted he could not have gotten a better training anywhere else. He said he felt confident he could handle practically any client situation without supervision. He was reminded that addiction has many faces and that each client comes to treatment with some degree of variance from all others. He was further encouraged to use consultation (one of a good counselor's 12 core functions) whenever a unique situation presents itself. Pete was assigned to work with Mario.

Mario's Story

Mario was a 21-year old male who had been using marijuana since he was 14 years old. About a year before enrolling in the Job Corps program, he began using methamphetamine. His drug test result indicated the presence of 230 nanograms of THC per millimeter of his blood and about 25,000 nanograms of methamphetamine. Within 52 hours of last usage, Mario was sitting in the counseling office with Pete undergoing as thorough an as assessment as Pete wanted it to be. Mario was saturated with drugs in his blood. As the THC and methamphetamine metabolites went to work, Mario was undergoing a rapid withdrawal. After nearly one hour of answering questions related to personal and family drug use history, Mario ran out of the counseling room and headed to his vocational counselor's office. He told his vocational counselor, Cindy, that he figured out what Job Corps was all about. He said the Job Corps program was a government conspiracy with the FBI to arrest and brain wash innocent weed smokers. He said he thought he recognized Pete as the same guy who arrested his father two years ago.

Pete paged the TEAP Specialist, who was in a meeting that afternoon and reported that Mario had taken off. Almost simultaneously, Cindy also paged. "You got one of those in my office. Come and get your boy before we loose him," Cindy said. Cindy had been with the program for a long time and has witnessed a variety of client problems. She offered Mario a hand full of snicker bars and told Mario that if there was one person in the world he could trust, it was the TEAP Specialist. Moments later the TEAP Specialist was finishing off the assessment with Mario. He told Mario that he (Mario) was very intelligent and even more so, very observant. He told Mario there was something about marijuana smokers that made them seem extremely smart. Mario began running his mouth in ignorance on how he made straight A(s) in school, smoking marijuana. He said he was getting ready to sign a record deal because marijuana helps him write and sing beautiful music. The TEAP Specialist told him that Pete had worked for several organizations before coming to Job Corps. He told Mario that since Pete is now a counselor, he has taken an oath to maintain confidentiality in all his dealings with clients. He was assured that he could trust Pete, no matter what his past career was. Six weeks into the program, we were laughing with Mario, in group therapy, about his psychotic suspicion of Pete working for FBI. Interestingly, Mario was asked to bring in some of the songs he recorded under the influence of marijuana for group review. When he returned from a weekend outing the following week, he brought back some of his self-recorded rap songs. The group had a good laugh with Mario over what he thought was a beautiful music under the influence of marijuana. The important thing to remember here is to not engage youth in lengthy assessment, especially during the initial assessment. As was mentioned in earlier chapters, the marijuana that youths use today is very potent. This means that youths generally are detoxifying from the drug for up to three weeks after they discontinue use. During the early detox, youths suffer shorter attention span, have neurotransmitters running wild in their brains, feel irritable, hallucinate, and feel paranoia. This is no time for prolonged assessment.

YOUTHS IN TREATMENT WANT TO BE IN 'CONTROL'

Many youths detest the idea of adults trying to control their lives. Freedom is one of our society's most valued inheritances. Freedom is enshrined in our constitution. We are taught to be assertive and many commercials urge us to take control of our lives. Part of our freedom right is the protection of our privacy, another provision of our constitution. Initial assessment for drug use can be invasive. A good counselor brings to the assessment table a tool kit full of assessment and diagnostic tools, ranging from the Alcohol Use Inventory, Alcohol Expectancy Questionnaire, Addiction Severity Index, to Substance Abuse Subtle Screening Inventory, Minnesota Multiphase Personality Inventory-2, the Millon Clinical Multiaxial Inventory-II, and Diagnostic and Statistical Manuel, Fourth Edition, to mention but a few. These tools generally tend to ask probing questions that tamper on a person's privacy. Many youths in treatment use drugs, among other things, because drug use denotes defiance to authority and an illusion of control over their own social lives. Assessment allows a counselor to develop a diagnostic evaluation of the client's substance abuse and any coexisting conditions in order to provide an integrated approach to treatment planning based on the client's strengths, weaknesses, and identified problems and needs. To do this effectively, a counselor will have to rely on the feedback from client and if the opportunity avails, feedback from client's immediate family members and/or friends. The diagnostic evaluation is the starting point for the development of the client's treatment plan. Within the assessment report, a counselor specifies a client's strengths and weaknesses in a comprehensive manner so that any member of the treatment team or future referral source would have a clear picture of the client's problem. Detailing the client's problems and needs is necessary in order to design intervention and treatment activities focused on the client's problem(s). This critical function of the counselor may be impeded, if the counselor does not maintain control of the interview techniques and assessment procedure. Indeed, if adequate therapeutic alliance is not developed with the client, assessment can be a frustrating experience for the beginning counselor. The situation can be exacerbated when working with youths, since youths tend to want to be in control.

In most social model recovery programs, it is emphasized that counselors confront inconsistencies when doing assessment with clients. Social model recovery programs may use group coercion during initial interview to subdue resistant clients into admission of substance use/abuse. Such techniques will drive a youth away from treatment. During the initial assessment with a youth, it may be necessary to allow inconsistent statements to go unchallenged or even allow a youth to remain in denial of her/his addiction. In other words, the counselor may have to be a "sucker' to the youth as part of the tactics in establishing therapeutic alliance. Debbie, who had worked for a social model recovery treatment center during the first phase of her internship, learnt different when she was assigned to do assessment on one of the Job Corps youth - Jason.

Jason's Story

Jason was 20 years old when he came to the Job Corps program. He had been using marijuana since he was 13 years old. He tested positive for marijuana (215ng/ml) and amphetamine (368ng/ml) on entry into the program. During the initial assessment he told Debbie he had never used drugs in his life and that no one in his family has ever used drugs. He said he went to a private school, where none of his friends used drugs. Debbie knew he was lying and had no problem challenging his contention. Debbie told Jason that the Job

Corps drug testing result is accurate because the drug test chain of custody does not allow for error. She told him that the drug-testing laboratory uses sophisticated equipments to perform the drug test. Jason became very angry. He immediately accused Debbie of calling him a liar and demanded to speak with the director of the program. Debbie told him he could not just speak to the director. She told him he could speak to the Health and Wellness Manager. Jason raised his voice loud and demanded to speak with some supervisor. He told Debbie she had no business calling him and 'his family' liars. He was adding dimension to the conflict every minute that passes. What started off as a private meeting inside the counseling office was now outside the office, while a crowd of Job Corps student watched Jason raise hell. He was enjoying every minute of the drama, because it gave him control of the situation.

A few minutes after, the TEAP Specialist arrived. He asked Jason and Debbie to step into the office. He demanded what happened. Jason immediately took charge and said Debbie called him and his family liars, because he told her that they have never used drugs. There was no sense in asking Debbie what happened, because there was nothing novel about the incident. It was a common occurrence for those who work with youths. Jason was told, much to Debbie's surprise, that even though the Job Corps urine specimen chain of custody was very fool proof, the lab had been known to make mistakes, including switching specimens. He told Jason he believed him. Jason demanded an apology from Debbie. The TEAP Specialist rejected the motion and took the blame. He told Jason it was his fault because he was supposed to read him the drug test result and not Debbie. He then apologized to Jason. He told Jason that even though the drug test result may be wrong, the Department of Labor (DOL funds the Job Corps training program) program regulation requires that the student be enrolled in the treatment program anyway, since the test result was positive. He told Jason: "you know the damn lab is not going to agree they made a mistake. I tell you what I'll do, since you've never used drugs, I'll just make you my assistant. You can help me treat these other guys who really have problems. Here, fill out these papers," he handed Jason the Addiction Severity Index assessment tool. Debbie was stunned at the TEAP Specialist approach. He told Jason to apologize to Debbie for embarrassing her, when all she tried to do was carry out her assigned duty. The TEAP Specialist also added that he knew Debbie would never call him a liar. Very softly Jason said she did not call her a liar, but doubting him was like calling him a liar. Again, the TEAP Specialist asserted that Debbie did not doubt him, but was instead explaining to him that the drug test procedure was foolproof from the test site level. Jason then apologized. During the second appointment with Jason, he admitted using drugs. He said he wanted to protect his parents who really had serious drug problem. He said he knew that in course of the treatment, it would be obvious that his parents use drugs, so he was basically trying to protect them. This is one of numerous denial mechanisms among youths and adult substance abusers. Weeks into treatment Debbie successfully challenged every inconsistency in Jason's drug use history. Ninety days into treatment Jason was telling a newcomer in the group "denial is not a river in Egypt. It is real. Right Doc?" he'll say to the TEAP Specialist.

Initial assessment must also take into consideration the cultural background of youths from both ethnic and social standpoint. Drug abuse and involvement has a disproportionate impact on the health and wellbeing of racial/ethnic minority communities evidenced by such indicators as increased drug-related illnesses such as HIV/AIDS, children living in foster care or with grandparents and crime infested neighborhoods. Youth sub-cultures are also impacted as evidenced by a growing number of rave parties, gang activities, school dropouts and youth crimes. The National Institute on Drug Abuse (NIDA) published a treatment research summary containing thirteen principles in 1999. The fourth principle specifically states that the treatment approach be appropriate to the individual's ethnicity and culture. The director of NIDA states that "addiction is treatable if well delivered and tailored to the particular patient within a cultural context." The director of the Center for Substance Abuse Treatment emphasizes, the critical role that cultural perspective contributes to treatment efficacy. Suggestions are offered for how individual counselors can improve competency in working with clients from racial/ethnic communities:
1. Objectively analyze your ability to offer culturally competent care to youths. Knowledge of culture both ethnic and social, especially

sub-cultures are essential. 2. Involve youths in the program implementation and review. Encourage youths to share ideas that contribute to program effectiveness, and learn from youths in the process. 3. Understand how race/ethnicity may affect therapeutic interactions and treatment programs. Pinderhughes (1989) in her book, *Understanding Race, Ethnicity, and Power*, states that experiences related to cultural differences can lead to internalizations, which can cause clients to misperceive or distort the intensions and interventions of practitioners. It is, therefore, crucial for the therapist to fully appreciate and attend to the many ways in which these perceptions and power issues enter and affect the therapeutic process. 4. Be open to difficult conversations about race, racism, prejudice, discrimination and cultural heritage. 5. Do not over generalize from one client to another. Although persons share a common overall culture, there is great diversity within populations. 6. Ask for help. Sources include colleagues, professional associations, churches and other clients – anyone who is likely to have answer. And 7. Have information and resources available. Try to have onsite public information that is culturally and linguistically appropriate.

On the average, African American male youths do not feel comfortable talking about their family, especially parents, in treatment setting. By contrast, African American female youths will very easily talk about their family, but will conceal information about their own personal family abuse. Further, African American male youths are apprehensive about how information divulged in counseling will be used. Many fear such information may be reported to law enforcement or will be used against them for employment purposes.

Jovon's Story

In working with a young African American male client (Jovon) from the Job Corps program, it became obvious that initial assessment will need a unique approach. Jovon was 18 years old when he arrived at the program. Like many youths, he had been using marijuana and alcohol since eight grade. His mother abused crack cocaine for as long as he could remember. His father was an alcoholic, who left his mother when Jovon was 13 years old. Jovon came to the program with a lot of anger. During initial assessment he was asked if any of his family member used drugs. "Why you got to bring my family into this? I don't appreciate people talking about my family," he said. His voice was loud. He spoke with clenched fist. The veins on his forehead popped up and his lips were tight. "Wow, my bad, said the TEAP Specialist. I don't even know why I asked. This aint about your family. Please disregard that question." Jovon appears visibly angry at the mention of his family, thereby calling for a refocus on his assessment. The tactics used on Jovon was to talk about his "road dogs or dawgs" (close friends). A wise mother once said: "show me your friend and I will tell you who you are." Jovon spent 30 minutes talking about how he was never home. He said he spent most of his time at his friend's house playing video games. He said his friend's mom was a "crack head" (crack cocaine abuser) and that his dad was in the "pen" (penitentiary). This meant that they (Jovon and his friend) basically fended for themselves. He said they "hustled" (sold drugs) daily to make ends meet. Few weeks after, it was clear that everything Jovon said about his friend's parents and more was actually about his own parents. It turned out that Jovon had a lot of anger directed at his parents, whom he said were never there for him.

Shanika's Story

On the other hand, a female African American client (Shanika) had no problem talking about her parents during initial assessment. When asked how she started using drugs, she began crying and would not say anything else. The initial assessment was ended on the note that she was very beautiful and sounded quiet intelligent. Those last deliberately planted comments kept her anxious to return for the second assessment. The TEAP Specialist has had experience working with Shanika's type – young African American female youths who had been sexually molested by a family member. Physical, verbal and sexual abuse is a common occurrence among African American female youths from single parent and underprivileged families. During the second assessment, Shanika admitted that nobody ever told her she was beautiful. She was reassured that she was and by the end of the session, she had told about how two of her mom's ex-boy friends had sexually molested her over a three year span. Child abuse report was sent out to the Department of Child Protective Services, because she was only seventeen years old at the time of treatment.

There is the issue of trust among African American male youths. Historically, they seem to not trust the "system." Years of historical oral tradition passed down from preceding generations reinforce subliminal messages that the "Whiteman" wants them to fail, and that the ultimate goal of white America is to put all black people in jail. The unsuspecting counselor will have problem getting to the presenting problem when an African American youth comes to treatment. Even when the counselor is African American, there seems to be the general notion that such a counselor has sold out to the system and therefore cannot be trusted. An African American male youth once told his African American counselor that he wont understand his plight because he (the counselor) had sold out and now has his fancy tie, clean car and nice job. "How can you help me? You never lived in my kind of neighborhood where cops are after you 24/7, and helicopter fly over your roof all night trying to put a brother in jail." He was talking to a veteran counselor who stopped him short on his sniveling: "I've been there, done that, "f" that," the counselor said. "All I'm trying to do is show you how you can get out of that madness. Now you can take it or go on back out there and find yourself a permanent address in jail. It's up to you. What are you going to do?" That was the turning point for that particular youth. The Substance Abuse and Mental Health Services Administration's (SAMHSA) Center for Substance Abuse (CSAT) released a report in 1999 on the critical role that cultural perspective plays in successful substance abuse treatment strategies. The report provides background on demographics, social and treatment needs for:

- African American (church support)
- Hispanic, (well-educated professionals may not understand the problems and cultural nuances of a poor immigrant community)
- Asian American/Pacific Islander (behavior labeled dysfunctional or enabling in the majority population is seen as appropriate protection of the individual)

- American Indian/Alaska Native populations (the community must be included in the treatment process and tribal healers, elders and holy persons must serve as counselors and support staff0

The report shows that some substance-abuse problems are more prevalent among some racial and ethnic minority populations and that members of these populations are disproportionately affected by diseases associated with alcohol and drugs abuse, such as HIV/AIDS, cirrhosis and other liver diseases, hepatitis and sexually transmitted diseases. Ignoring these factors, the report warns, can lead to a one-size-fits-all mentality that may set the stage for more costly and acute treatment needs down the road. Culturally competent services, among other things, must include:

1. Staff knowledge of the native language or vernacular of the cultural group
2. Staff sensitivity of the cultural nuances of the patient population (recent immigrants do have the same experiences as earlier arrivals)
3. Staff backgrounds may benefit from representation of those of the patient population
4. Treatment modalities that reflect the cultural values and treatment needs of the patient population (i.e. incorporating American Indian rituals, Pacific Islander rituals, or Hispanic family dynamics into the treatment program)
5. Representation of the patient population in decision-making and policy implementation so outsiders are not imposing their values.

The above-mentioned may seem far-fetched, but a close examination of a real case scenario makes the case. One of the female Caucasian counselors (Paula) was once working with a Hispanic youth (Armando), who was a third generation gangster from South Central, Los Angeles.

Armando's Story

Armando was referred to the Job Corps program by his probation officer as a final resort to keep him out of the streets and out of trouble, for good. Armando tested positive for marijuana on entry into the program. He proudly declares his gang affiliation and claims he has been using drugs since he was five years old. He said his dad used to get him drunk when he was 10 years old. During assessment Paula wanted to know whom Armando lived with prior to entering the program. Armando informed her that he lived with his grandmother, but that he spent most of his time in the streets. As part of determining the family drug use history Paula asked Armando if her grandmother uses drugs. Armando went ballistic. While Hispanic grandmothers, like the grandmothers of any other race may possibly use drugs, the Hispanics have a very high regard for their grandmothers. In fact, the grandmother is the unspoken head of the household in a Hispanic family. Armando said Paula had disrespected him. He called her profane names and demanded an apology. Paula, in turn, reasoning that she had done nothing clinically wrong attempted to explain to Armando her reason for asking the question, but Armando was in no mood to hear her. Following series of offensive name calling from Armando, Paula lost her composure and added insult to injury when she told Armando she was not scared of his gang affiliation. In the heat of the argument that ensued, the TEAP Specialist emerged to save the day. "Say, homes, you're right. Nobody should talk about anybody's grandmother like that," said the TEAP Specialist. "Tell this B—h that," Armando said. "Wow, wow, wow, we're not going to call people names, homes," the TEAP Specialist ordered. "She started it," Armando said. The TEAP Specialist told Armando he was a leader and that leaders have to show good example. He told Armando that a lot of youths in the program would be looking up to him, because of his vast experiences. Armando took the flattery well. In a few minutes Armando apologized to Paula and we were on our way to treatment planning. Armando remained a challenge for several weeks before his moment of awakening. In the meanwhile Paula learned to be sensitive about approaching grandmother issues when working with certain group.

Azuka's Story

Another case involved an African youth. Generally, you do not see many Africans in treatment. Many Africans have core values that provide resiliency to substance abuse in foreign lands Azuka was 23 years old when he arrived to treatment. He said his parents had warned him not to go to America, but he did not listen. He came to America under a government scholarship program. Azuka had been to two other treatment programs before his elder brother brought him to the Job Corps program. He seems to have entrapped himself in a self-fulfilling prophecy. He believed his parents had cursed him and that the gods will never forgive him for using marijuana and cocaine until the curse was lifted. In fact, he strongly believed that the reason he used drugs, in the first place, was because of the curse. After a relapse within three weeks of enrollment in the program, the TEAP Specialist had to resort to unorthodox measure. He consulted with a colleague who also was African. A special ritualistic counseling was arranged for Azuka. The colleague arrived, posing as a chief from the same tribe as Azuka. He brought with him a special brand of gin. He then proceeded to undo the curse, after communicating to the gods and pouring the gin on the ground for the gods. He took some mud and rubbed across Azuka's forehead, rebuking the curse and invoking nothing but goodness and mercy. Azuka completed the program without another relapse. He finished his vocational training and left the Job Corps program with a job.

The fore going vignettes are only a snap shot of some of the dynamics that come into interplay when working with youths. The focus of this section of this book is not to examine cultural influences in working with youths, but instead, to highlight them as part of the dynamics that make it difficult to sometimes come across to youths. One African American counselor intern once challenged a 16-year-old Korean youth when she reported she had not used drugs during a follow-up counseling. The counselor intern said she knew the girl was lying because she did not have eye contact when she answered the question. Later, the intern counselor learned that most Asians do not maintain eye contact as a sign of respect, especially to someone in authority or to seniors. What is important is that parent, teachers, significant adults and counselors understand that working with youths require creativity and sometimes unusual approach. Youth themselves present unusual perspective to life. It becomes imperative to be fully equipped when working with them. Youths tend to rebel when adults try to "control" their lives. Working with youths requires that one speak to them on the same level. For counselors, it is important not to engage in clinical talk. Clinical talk may come across to youth the same way they view adult talk. They get the impression they are at fault. They are bad and need to change. Change is something most youths feel they are not ready for. Many times counselor interns bring a youth in the counseling office and announce to the youth that she/he tested positive for 250 nanograms of marijuana. The youth becomes suddenly apprehensive at this seemingly judgmental disclosure of drug test result. The youth raises the iron curtain of denial or at the very least assume a confrontational position, because implicit in the drug test result is the underlying tone of "you are bad." The TEAP Specialist brings a youth into the office and casually says: "Men, you must have been smoking some good 'chronic' or 'endo,' because your drug test result was off the hook." In other words, your urinalysis came back with high nanograms of tetrahydrocannabinol. This approach usually takes the youth by surprise. Youths do not expect their adult counselor or therapist to talk like that. When they hear a counselor talk like that, they immediately assume that the adult "understands" and that she/he is "cool;" They also tend to bond with the counselor, just by using their level of linguistic expression. By the way, "chronic" and "endo" are slang for hybrid marijuana. As parents, teachers and counselors we tend to not show interest in youth culture, which include their mode of expression. We fail to realize that it is only a phase that passes with time and age. Remember when you were a youth? Is it possible you used language the way your parents did not? When adults share youth's language, youths tend to be attracted to such adults. Now by no means do we mean to imply that an adult has to compromise her/his ethics, firmness, moral standing and integrity in the process of communicating with youths. As for counselors, you want to be your youth client's "friend" without being their friend. This simply means that you want to communicate with youths in such a way as to make them feel wanted, make them want to be your friend, make them feel they can trust you and actually show them you can be trusted, without fraternizing, personally socializing or compromising your counselor/client relationship. Obviously, this requires skill and practice. A young African American youth once decided he would not cooperate during assessment with one of the counselors. After two days of refusing to give details to any question other than those that required a yes or no answer, the TEAP Specialist was called in to help. The TEAP Specialist, who himself is African American, entered the room, looked the youth client straight in the eyes and said, "what's up player? Men, are those some Jordon? (He was referring to the client's tennis shows). Nigga that is tight." That was all it took. The youth who had refused to say a word in two days was now running his mouth explaining how much he paid for the Michael Jordon brand tennis show and how many points Jordon scored in basketball during the season. One hour after, the youth was crying about how he had been neglected by his drug-using parents who abandoned him three years ago, and how he had to sell drugs to survive. As was stated earlier, these short illustrations were taken from real live counseling situation. The client's real names have been changed for obvious reasons. So far, we have been very permissive in dealing with youths during preliminary assessment. As most counselors know, assessment is on going and the counselor has to strive to keep up with changing mood of the youth throughout the counseling process. In chapter five we will take a tougher stance with the youth client without destroying the therapeutic alliance that was developed during the initial assessment. All inconsistency noted during the initial assessment will be confronted during individual counseling. We will learn how to convince a youth that she/he can benefit from treatment. We will also learn how to uncover the emotional injury, which is known to be the forerunner of substance abuse in many youths. We will then examine specific treatment approaches that have proven useful in working with youths. As with the previous chapters will use case situations to illustrate the effectiveness of chosen treatment approaches.

CHAPTER FIVE

INDIVIDUAL COUNSELING:
THE FIRST LINE OF OFFENSE IN WORKING
WITH YOUTHS

Counseling entails the utilization of special skills to assist individuals or group in resolving their presenting problems. Youths tend to favor individual counseling in the early phase of treatment. Each youth feel unique about her/his problem and therefore, seem to prefer dealing with issues in private. Group counseling is equally effective, however, individual counseling allows the youth to groom for group participation later in treatment. The counseling process strives to resolve problems through exploration and ramifications of presenting and anecdotal issues and consideration of alternative solutions. Cognitive, behavioral and affective factors are examined with a view to changing or improving decision making. Competency is required in order to prevent causing additional injury to a client. Practitioners often try to delineate the difference between counseling and psychotherapy. E.F. Borgatta and W.W. Lambert (1968) contend they are the same qualitatively, but they differ only quantitatively. "I realized some years ago that there was nothing that a psychotherapist did that a counselor did not do," (Corsini, 1968). E.F. Borgatta and W.W. Lambert used the table below to depict the quantitative difference between counseling and psychotherapy. They believe there is no fundamental difference between counseling and psychotherapy:

Estimation of Percentage of Time Spent by Counselors and Psychotherapists in Professional Activities.

PROCESS	COUNSELING	PSYCHOTHERAPY
Listening	20	60
Questioning	15	10
Evaluation	5	5
Interpreting	1	3

Supporting	5	10
Explaining	15	5
Informing	20	3
Advising	10	3
Ordering	9	1

Corsini purports that no definition can be made which will include all counseling methods. He maintains that the various attempts to separate the psychotherapies and exclude all counseling methods have failed. He further added that the concept that psychotherapy goes into depth while counseling does not is gainsaid by such procedures as behavior modification, which operates at the level of symptoms removal. In his view, behavior modifiers could hardly be called counselors, because they do not counsel. "And when we have a term such as nondirective counseling, we have a semantic absurdity if we think about it long enough. In this book, counseling and therapy will be used interchangeably. For example when we talk about developing therapeutic alliance, we might as well be referring to a counseling alliance with a client. The counseling process establishes a relationship between a counselor and her or his client. Effective counseling facilitates clients' problem identification, attitudes and value modification, and behavior changes. The effective counselor bases his or her counseling on an examination of alternative solutions to the presenting problem of the client and the client's active involvement in decision-making.

All counseling techniques are methods of learning, which are intended to change people: to make them think differently (cognition), to make them feel differently (affection), and to make them act differently (behavior). Indeed, counseling is learning: It may be learning something new or re-learning something one has forgotten; it may be learning how to learn or it may be unlearning; paradoxically, it may even be learning what one already knows. Let's examine closely the three modes of counseling:

Cognition – There are two general ways we learn. We can learn thing directly by experience or indirectly through symbols. For example, a 13-year-old boy goes into his parents' liquor cabinet and helps himself to a full cup of vodka and drinks it all up. We will assume that this 13-year-old boy has never drunk alcohol of any kind before. The boy gets intoxicated, vomits all over himself and gets a serious scolding, including grounding from several activities as a result. The boy would have learned several things experientially. Namely, drinking alcohol creates an uncomfortable feeling of intoxication; his parents do not approve of him drinking; drinking alcohol makes him loose his privileges and earns him disrespect from his parents. Another way the boy would have learned the same lessons would have been by symbols. His parents would have told him that drinking alcohol as a minor may lead to an embarrassing and uncomfortable feeling of drunkenness, which in turn, will cause him to loose certain privileges. In both cases, the boy learns – in one case, actively (through experience) and in another case, passively (through information). Some counselors tend to use "active" methods and their clients essentially learn on their own, while some counselors tend to make their clients passive learners.

Behavior – Learning can occur through action. Physical fitness was part of the Job Corps substance abuse treatment for youths. Youths were made to carry out high-impact aerobic exercise and weight lifting. The modality of treatment component was plain physical exercise, which is believed to be psychotherapeutic by many. Such type of physical therapy teaches youth self-confidence, allows fatigue to set in for those who have problem sleeping because of marijuana detox, produces endorphins, which allows the youths to feel mild euphoria, and increases metabolites of tetrahydrocannabinol. Some may argue that body therapy does not include the mind. On the contrary, the mind does exist, because the condition of the body affects the mind. In other words, if we work from the outside in, by changing the body we can change the mind. As the youths change their bodies, they tend to like what they see and learn to respect their bodies. An analogy to the body and mind argument will be plastic surgery. Changing someone's looks can affect how that person views herself or himself. Other examples of physical behavior as psychotherapy would include complex physical activities, such as role playing, or doing therapeutic homework, that is, doing under direction things one would not ordinarily do, such as asking for a date or looking for job. As in the case of cognitive therapies, behavioral work in therapy can range from active to passive.

Affection – Many substance abuse counselors work more with the affective component of psychotherapy, popularly known as emotions or feelings. We cannot really work directly with the emotions and must reach them indirectly through the intellect or the body. Consequently, we cannot manipulate emotions in the sense that we can manipulate thinking or behaving. Some systems of psychotherapy are intended to reduce or negate emotions, seeing them as hindering the therapeutic process. Adlerian psychotherapy, for example, is essentially a cognitive therapy, and Adlerians usually see emotions as sabotaging efforts in the therapeutic process. However, in psychodrama, for example, both the words that the therapist will employ and the behavior directed by the other actors are intended to generate strong emotions. Some people see emotions as epiphenomena accompanying but affecting therapeutic change, while others see emotions as a powerful agent leading to change and still others see emotions as evidence of change. The whole issue of the relationship of emotions to psychotherapy is unsettled.

All therapies are essentially combinations of all three of these modalities. While some are rather pure in that they attempt to deal only with the body, the intellect, or the emotions, elements of each apply in most cases. Thus, for example, in Rational-Emotive Therapy, even though rational thinking is utilized for the most part in dealing with the patient, the therapist may suggest to the client to do certain things (homework) and thus there will be a strong behavioral component. And in cognitive therapy such as Transactional Analysis, emotionally upsetting situations will develop. A therapist may think that improvement is a function of one element, but the curative process may actually be something else. It may not be a message that generated a change, but rather the interpretation that the client gives to being handled. That means that change may well result from the interpretation, "someone cares for me enough to do this for me." One final common pathway for all therapies is a new way of seeing life, a reevaluation of self and others. If so, then all therapies are essentially cognitive. Still another way of considering psychotherapy is to see it as a process of "selling" – of trying to help a person to accept a new view of self and of others. From this point of view the psychotherapist is a persuader or a facilitator in attempting to change opinions. In order to motivate people to change, it is important to understand the mechanisms and elements of therapy. Corsini and Rosenberg (1955) identified nine factors embedded in the three modes of psychotherapy discussed earlier – Cognitive, Behavioral and Affective factors.

Cognitive Factors
- *Universality.* Clients improve when they realize that they are not alone, that others have similar problems, and that human suffering is universal.
- *Insight.* Growth occurs as clients increasingly come to understand themselves and others and gain different perspective on their own motives and behavior.
- *Modeling.* People benefit from watching other people. In group therapy both the counselor and other group members may serve as models.

Behavioral Factors
- *Reality testing.* Change becomes possible when clients experiment with new behaviors in the safety of the therapy hour, receiving support and feedback from the counselor and other group members.
- *Ventilation.* This factor encompasses those statements attesting to the value of "blowing off steam" through shouting, crying, or displaying anger in a context in which one could still feel accepted.
- *Interaction.* Clients improve when they are able to openly admit to the group that there is something wrong with themselves or their behavior.

Affective Factors
- *Acceptance.* This factor reflected the sense of being part of the group and getting unconditional positive regard, especially from the counselor.

- *Altruism.* Change can result from the recognition that one is the recipient of the love and care of the counselor or other members of the group or from being the one who provides love and care to others.
- *Transference.* This factor identifies the emotional bond that occurs between the counselor and the client or between clients in a group setting.

Corsini believes these nine factors encapsulate the basic mechanisms of therapeutic change. Close examination of these models, he said, reveals that the cognitive factors imply "Know yourself,' the affective factors tell us "Love your neighbor," and the behavioral factors essentially suggest, "Do good work." The modes and factors of psychotherapy are accomplished using one or more of various counseling techniques: Rational Emotive Therapy, Rational Behavioral Therapy, Cognitive Therapy, Reality Therapy, Transactional Analysis, to mention but a few. We will examine some of these methods in chapter six. For now, we will examine specific techniques used in directing youths to change.

CONFRONTING INCONSISTENCIES AND CONNECTING DOTS

In chapter four we emphasized that a counselor, teacher, parent, mentor or significant adult working with marijuana impaired youth should not confront inconsistencies during the initial assessment interview with the youth. We also said it was imperative that we develop treatment or therapeutic alliance with the youth. Once an alliance is properly developed, it becomes necessary to confront denial, inconsistencies and maladaptive or self-defeating behavior. We learn to pull together, the youth's fragmented view of her/his presenting problem, thereby allowing the youth to see connection between marijuana abuse and personal failure. Once the youth is able to see that there is a direct correlation between marijuana abuse and social, psychological, economical and/or legal problems the youth encounter, only then is the youth ready to give treatment a fair chance. For the counselor, the ability to "connect dots' means that

76

once therapeutic alliance is established, the counselor, parent, mentor or significant adult must role model certain personal qualities: enthusiasm, sincerity, openness, honesty, trust-worthiness and self respect. They also need to demonstrate unconditional positive regard and respect for the youth, and relate to the youth with flexibility, open-mindedness, and optimism, while displaying firmness and expecting accountability. The youth must be seen as a unique individual, who needs an individualized treatment plan. The youth worker must practice self-examination and deal with personal unresolved issues, which may interfere with professional effectiveness. The counselor's vast experiences when used with care and diligence will foster youth's cognitive, behavioral and affective coping skills, which work together to activate the change process.

Confronting inconsistencies the youth presented during assessment requires skills and sound counseling techniques such as listening actively. This means that one not only listen for content, but also interpret process, referring to the youth's non-verbal cues, such as facial expressions. Empathy (attempting to understand the youth's feelings, while maintaining objectivity and a separate sense of self) is another effective technique. The counselor probes youths by asking open-ended questions ('what' and 'how'), which invite broader responses and thereby allows the counselor to explore new leads into the presenting problem. Clarifying and paraphrasing responses helps the counselor reflect feeling and content back to the youth in a "here and now" manner, using timely, accurate, fair, objective and descriptive feedback. This promotes additional understanding of the problem by emphasizing immediacy. For example, the counselor may call attention to the fact that because the youth spent too much time hanging out with his friends who smoke marijuana, the youth did not devote enough time to job search and therefore, missed out on important job opportunities. Further, the counselor is able to engage in making skilled interpretations, when appropriate, and using descriptive confrontation, which involves stating mainly facts and not opinion. For example, a youth once claimed that he has never used drugs before, despite the fact his test result came back positive for marijuana. The counselor agreed with him, but then asked: "Can you think of how marijuana smoke got into your blood." The youth responded by suggesting that it might have been through 'contact high' with his cousin who spokes marijuana regularly. The counselor knew at that point that the youth was up to some deceit. First of all, the counselor reasoned, the fact the youth knows about 'contact high' (experiencing euphoria by being exposed to thick smoke of marijuana over a very long period of time) means that he knows a lot about drug use; something a non-drug using youth might not know about. Secondly, the test result had a very high amount of THC in the youth's blood – more than scientifically feasible to be received through contact high. The counselor, again, responded: "You are right. It is possible to test positive through contact high. Just how long were you with your cousin while he smoked and where did this happen?" The youth said they were in his cousin's back yard for about one hour the night before he left for the Job Corps program. As if to appear innocent he added he was trying to talk his cousin to stop using marijuana and join him to enter the Job Corps program. The counselor listened attentively and finally told the youth: "Your drug test result is so high that you would have to be in 4' by 8' room full of marijuana smoke, with no ventilation, for at least four hours in order for your drug test result to be so high from contact high." The youth laughed and said the truth was that his cousin always influenced him to use marijuana. Such is the extraneous length a counselor would have to go, sometimes, in order to extract the truth from youths in denial. Joan and Arden Christen (1990) offer guidelines that enhance client/counselor relationships:

- Join with client to plan mutually agreed upon treatment goals
- Use a gentle and courteous "carefronting," not an abrasive, confronting approach
- Avoid labeling clients or their problems with judgmental, evaluative language; instead, use descriptive terms
- Be prepared to alter the treatment approach, as each client's therapeutic status changes
- Lead, don't push, clients toward self-knowledge; position them to discover personal truths, don't merely supply the 'right' answers

- Avoid overusing certain techniques and remember that no technique can ever replace honest concern and emphatic support
- Show balance in your approach; never demand total compliance, but set limits and expect accountability
- Determine what stage of pre-recovery or recovery each client is in and plan accordingly
- Consider the type of problem that the client is dealing with, in planning treatment. (Addiction problems necessitate active, directive interventions and vigorous follow-up procedure
- Evaluate each client's personal characteristics, in planning a treatment approach. I.e., Is the client verbal and highly cognitive? An educational approach, using teaching material, decision-making, problem solving, etc., may work well with this individual. Is the recovering client action-oriented? Assertion-training, contracting, reinforcement, etc., may be a good choice for him/her. Is the person non-verbal, passive, defensive, resistant or considerably younger than the counselor? Action-directive leadership may be more effective with anyone who display's these characteristics
- Use multiple intervention, whenever possible
- Encourage self-forgiveness and self-acceptance, when relapses occur; re-define these set backs as learning experiences; a part of the recovery process which provides new insights
- Accept each individual's recovery pace; do not impose your expectations onto clients
- Remind clients that recovery is volitional; explore 'pay-offs' for remaining addicted
- Reinforce the idea those who follow a well-planned, well executed, supportive and on-going therapeutic program can recover
- Emphasize the importance of the client in recovery, not merely the recovery goal.

The counselor needs to understand and tolerate the meaning behind client silences. These long pauses may seem to be (and sometimes are), signs of mistrust, fear, apathy or boredom. More likely, however, they represent the client's need to contemplate, and emotionally process 'here and now' issues. An effective counselor seeks to understand this phenomenon and use it therapeutically. Finally, the wise counselor also guards against excessive self-disclosure, a behavior that diminishes professional power. Counselors, who find themselves inappropriately seeking client's acceptance, through counter-transference or other means will wisely seek therapy themselves, where they can have their needs met as members, and not leaders, (Christen, 1990).

An effective counselor is like a detective, who examines all evidence in detail, corroborates all information and finding, arranges events in chronological sequence and connects all dots to determine what happened. In working with a youth, a good counselor must strive to piece all the bits of information the youth supplies together in order to determine the underlying causes or catalyst of addiction. Denial will most often blur and hinder the efforts of a counselor, but the experienced counselor, like a detective, knows how to separate fact from fiction. The detective looks for motive and opportunity, while a youth counselor looks for childhood or adolescence emotional injury, predisposition to addiction and socio-cultural environmental factors that precipitated and fueled on-set of addiction. Unearthing the underlying cause of the on-set of addiction can be difficult when working with youths. Oftentimes, some of the cultural issues mentioned earlier make it even more challenging. Such was the case with an African American youth, Stanley.

Stanley's Story

Stanley tested positive for marijuana and phencyclidine (PCP) on entry into the Job Corps system. He denied ever using PCP, but acknowledged he had a couple of puffs off a blunt (marijuana stick rolled with tobacco leaf) his cousin was smoking as a gesture of send off party, because he was leaving for Job Corps the next morning. The truth of the situation is that he had enough THC in his blood to get two more people high for two hours. That was all the information he was willing to divulge, since he does not "feel comfortable speaking to strangers about his problem." He denied using tobacco or alcohol and refused to talk about his family, claiming his family has nothing to do with him testing positive for marijuana. We completed the initial assessment within thirty minutes. He was asked to return for follow-up assessment in two days. During our second meeting, he was rather very quiet, preferring to say very little. The TEAP Specialist decided to break his silence by bringing up an issue that seemingly had nothing to do with the reason why he was there. "You scored very high on your entry tests. You must have attended a very good school or your family really helped you a lot when you were in school. Which one is it?" He appeared bewildered by the question. He leaned forward as though he wanted to say something, but changed his mind. His lips got tight and he silently clenched his fist. "Well, let me guess. Your dad used to help you. It was always my dad who used to help me," the TEAP Specialist said. That did it. "I don't want to talk about my f—kin parents," he yelled in a rage. "I'm sorry. I did not mean to offend you. Let's just talk about something else," the TEAP Specialist said: "You told me two days ago that you do not smoke cigarettes, nor drink alcohol, but I saw you smoking cigarette yesterday, after dinner, on my way home from work. But that's not all, you also told me you took a couple of puffs off your cousin's blunt the night before you arrived to the program. That is also not true, because your test result indicates you are either a regular user or you used heavily that one night. I want to believe the former, since you lied to me about smoking cigarettes. I am here to assist you put all these behind. It will be difficult for me unless you really want me to help you." Stanley was quiet. He threw his head down and said calmly: "It's easy for you to say how your dad used to help you study. I had to do it all by my self. I've been doing things for myself ever since I can remember. My mom cared more about her stupid husband and alcohol than to help me" At this point two issues had been identified; One, he was not getting along with his stepfather, and two, his mother is an alcoholic. "You called your father 'stupid husband.' Why is that?" Again, he clenched his fist in anger. His lips got tight and his eyes were squinted. "He is not my father," he said. "Where is your father?" He began his first honest attempt to tell his story: "My dad left my mother when I was three years old. I don't know my father. I don't have any good memory of him. My mom remarried when I was about six years old. Her husband never cared about my brother and me. I started smoking weed when I was in fourth grade and I have not stopped ever since. My mom must have started drinking after my dad left. That's all she does is drink all day. I started stealing her drink when I was eight. I just want to move on with my life." Stanley was 16 years old, soon to be 17, when this dialogue was taking place. He was assured that all would be well, if that is what he wants. He suddenly looked relieved, following his brief confession. It was possible that that was his first time talking about his life with anybody. He was asked to write down two good things about his stepfather and three good things about his mother that he remembers and bring it during the next meeting. He returned the next week with a list about his mother and nothing on his stepfather. He said he did not want to talk about his stepfather. Experience and counseling intuition preempted the situation. Stanley was told that he was not the first youth to be molested or abused by his stepfather, but holding back from talking about it would not help his case. He was assured that whatever the issue was, that it needed to be resolved, so he could move on with his life, like he said. Stanley began to weep. He said his stepfather had molested him when he was eight years old and the ordeal continued till he was nine. He said he told his mother that her husband touched him, but she defended him, so he never bothered to tell her after that. A child abuse report was sent to the child Protective Services and his treatment plan was modified to accommodate the new information. Notice how coincidental his molestation and the on-set of stealing his mother's alcohol, coupled with smoking marijuana at the age of nine were. One thing that stood out over the years in working with many youths that abuse drugs is that many have suffered serious abuse of some sort, whether it is physical, familial or emotional. These youths have been dubbed 'youths with wounded souls.' Emotional abuse on young people is usually a catalyst or precursor to substance abuse. Even more so, addiction appears to be trans-generational. That is, frequently addiction may have been modeled by older or deceased relatives and repeated in the next generation. This is why a counselor must try to ascertain family history of substance abuse during assessment.

Children who sustain emotional injuries carry their wounded souls through youth to adulthood. They often are reluctant to talk about their traumatic experiences. A good counselor learns to scout for these emotional injuries. Special skills are needed in this area. If the duration of treatment is short or the treatment modality calls for brief group interaction, perhaps, it may be a good idea for the counselor to refer the youth to an appropriate agency where adequate help will be received. Otherwise, the counselor opens up a gashing wound from the past, but merely puts a band-aid on it, instead of providing healing. This may cause the youth more harm. Scouting for emotional injury requires that the counselor become familiar with some of the characteristics of adult children of trauma. Robert J. Ackerman, Ph.D. identifies several characteristics:

- Learned Helplessness – A person loses the feeling that they can affect or change what is going on
- Depression – Unexpressed and unfelt emotion lead to flat internal world or agitated/anxious depression
- Emotionally Constricted – Numbness and shutdown as a defense against overwhelming pain and threat. Lack of range of expression or authentic expression of emotion
- Distorted Reasoning – Convoluted attempts to make reason out of senseless pain
- Loss of Trust and Faith – Due to deep rupture in primary, dependency relationships and breakdown of an orderly world
- Hyper Vigilance – Anxiety, waiting for the other shoe to drop; constantly scanning environment and relationships for signs of potential danger or repeated rupture
- Traumatic Bonding – Unhealthy bonding style resulting from power imbalance in relationships and lack of other sources of support
- Loss of Ability to Take in Support – Due to fear of trusting and depending upon relationships and emotional breakdown
- Loss of Ability to Modulate Emotion – Go from 0 to 10 and 10 to 0 without intermediate steps, rashness, loss of control, black and white thinking
- Easily Triggered – Stimuli reminiscent of trauma, e.g., yelling, loud noises, criticism, or gunfire, trigger person into shutting down, acting out or intense emotional states

- High Risk Behaviors – Speeding, sexual acting out, spending, fighting; jump starting inner world; acting out intense inner world
- Disorganized Inner World – Disorganized object constancy and relatedness; fused feelings (e.g., anger and sex)
- Survival Guilt – From witnessing abuse and trauma and surviving, from 'getting out' of a particular family system
- Development of Rigid Psychological Defenses – Dissociation, denial, splitting, withdrawal, aggression
- Cycle of Reenactment – Unconscious repetition of pain-filled dynamics
- Desire to self Medicate – Attempts to quiet and control turbulent, troubled inner world through the use of drugs and alcohol

Toxic shame is also associated with childhood trauma and often becomes the core of addiction. Fossum and Mason (1986) identify shame as the central force, which drives and intensifies addictive practices. Shame is differentiated from guilt in the following manner: guilt is behaviorally based; it is experienced when a person acts in a way, which violates her/his personal value system. That is, "I did something bad. I made a mistake." However, its' eventual outcome can be restitution, learning and growth. In contrast, personal shame is deep-seated sense of being an unworthy, invalid, defective human being with little or no chance for positive change and growth. That is, "I am bad. I am a mistake." Bradshaw (1989) makes a further distinction between toxic shame, an autonomous, destructive force, and healthy shame (realistic acknowledgement of one's human condition). Bradshaw describes toxic shame as a 'being' wound, a sense of total non-acceptance, which colors every relationship in which the shame-based person is involved. Many children raised in inappropriate guilt and shame-inducing family systems carry excessive, irrational, feelings of guilt and shame into adulthood. Now manifested in self-contempt, these feelings can prompt people to choose dysfunctional companions, chemical usage and other addictive escape mechanisms. Family shame is sustained by the 'no talk' rule, whereby past negative family events (e.g., suicide, tragic death, incest, sexual molestation, aberrant behaviors, crimes, etc.) continue to be hidden over the years. These dark family secrets emanates in the behavior of family members in various ways: overachieving, highly sensitive, fearful of conflict, inability to keep a healthy relationship, etc. Along with the tendencies to repress sensitive information, other characteristics of shame-based person and families include perfectionism, projection of blame, denial and resistance to change. Children who grow up within these restrictive parameters learn to manage life by developing superficial relationships and interactions, self-defeating, obsessive, compulsive, phobic or abusive behaviors and unhealthy ego. Once the counselor is able to uncover the emotional injury and connects the dots from the on-set of addiction to the youth's presenting problem, the counselor is ready to develop an appropriate treatment plan.

HEALING EMOTIONAL INJURIES

Emotional injuries are deep-seated. Oftentimes, they have been repressed for so long that the injured has learned unhealthy coping mechanisms to sooth the pain associated with the injury. Over a considerable period, the injured forms dysfunctional core values. The act of healing the emotionally injured youths calls for sound clinical practice, creativity, consistent intervention during various stages of treatment and ultimately instilling resiliency into the youth, once new coping skills have been set in place. Resiliency, the ability to thrive despite adversity, enables people of all ages and backgrounds to lead healthy and fulfilling lives despite formidable obstacles. So, how does a counselor move a youth from a position of utter hopelessness to hope, from denial to acceptance, from I can't succeed to I will try, from no one can help me to I think you can help me. An African proverb teaches: "He who is down need not fear falling." Many youths who come to treatment feel like they have nothing to loose. When people feel they have nothing to loose, they are usually unrestrained as to the amount of risk they are willing to take. They develop a defensive attitude toward others and sometimes towards their own selves. There is neither trust nor cooperation in dealing with others. In fact, there is a general spirit of 'them against us' and vice versa. To begin healing, the counselor must revisit the fundamental teaching of the African proverb cited above. The counselor must pick up the youth, offer the youth a crutch, or become the figurative human crutch. Once the youth feels a sense of balance, suddenly, the fear of falling returns. At this point, we are ready to begin healing. However, much will not be accomplished until the youth has been given the opportunity to unearth and relive the repressed event, understand what happened, understand her/his role or no role in what happened, accept the event as exactly what it is and make an effort to move on with life. This whole process can be painful. The process calls for scratching up old injuries, thereby, causing the youth to purge some emotion – an exercise commonly called catharsis or in more technical terms, abreaction.

Some experts in the field of psychotherapy decried the usefulness of emotional abreaction or catharsis (the release of tension and anxieties by reliving and unburdening those traumatic incidents which, in the past, were originally associated with the repression of the emotion) during the mid 50s to early 60s. That era saw the burgeoning of many forms of therapy in which the central focus of the treatment consisted of self-expression, releasing emotion, overcoming inhibitions, and articulating in speech and behavior the fantasies or impulses previously suppressed. The Encounter Movement (Burton, 1969; Schultz, 1967) represents one such school. Primal Scream Therapy is another. These forms of treatment represent exaggerations and caricatures of the principle of emotional catharsis that Sigmund Freud advanced in his early studies of hysteria. At that time, he thought that discharge of pent-up emotion could have a beneficial therapeutic effect. Subsequent experience with the treatment of neurotic patients, however, convinced Freud (1894) that this method was limited and, in the long run, ineffectual, since it did not give sufficient weight to the needs of self-punishment and various defenses the ego uses to ward off anxiety. Despite the shortcoming noted, catharsis/abreaction and confession may afford the client relief by freeing her/him from carrying the burden of "unfinished business." Beside, catharsis may also be a test of whether the client can place trust in the counselor. Catharsis involves the freeing of psychic energy that accompanies an expansion of consciousness. As the psyche includes previously disowned parts of itself, the energies previously exerted in the service of repression become available for more conscious utilization. In addition, there is a sense of relief in reuniting with an important part of the self that had been previously hidden or disowned. Moreno (1946-69) in his various work on psychodrama, using catharsis, noted that psychodrama aims not only at a rediscovery of the various aspects of the self, but also at developing constructive ways of utilizing these dimensions. Referring to this principle, Moreno noted that every catharsis of abreaction should be followed by a catharsis of integration. He cautions that therapies aimed simply at abreactive catharsis may have been less effective because they lack the component of developing healthy behaviors to replace the unhealthy ones. When people discover that they can be accepted by a group or find a meaningful role in the world, a catharsis of belonging occurs, which may also include spiritual or transpersonal experiences. The unique focus of psychodrama in encouraging the expansion of the self in a group setting creates an opportunity for synthesizing the needs for both individuation and belonging. By demanding a holistic involvement from the counselor, psychodrama functions not only as a method for developing insight, but also as a method of experiential learning, which facilitates personal growth for the counselor as well as the client. As was mentioned earlier, reliving and recounting painful emotions in the presence of a supportive, trusted ally (counselor) allows the youth to own and accept her/his feelings, thereby, permitting the youth to acknowledge affect-laden materials that were unconscious. The process, in turn, prepares the youth to drop her/his guards and become receptive to new ideas. So, how does the counselor harness the abreactive energy out of the youth? Recall that following resistance to divulge information, Stanley finally admitted his stepfather molested him. That was the turning point for Stanley, yet it was the beginning of a carefully structured series of steps of catharsis. Stanley had so far lived his youthful life under the "Unspoken Rules of Troubled Families," (Ackerman, 2002): Be in control at all times; Always be right, do the right thing; If something doesn't happen as planned, blame someone, yourself or another person; Deny feelings, especially the negative or vulnerable ones like

anxiety, fear, loneliness, grief, rejection or need; Don't expect
reliability or consistency in relationships; Don't bring transactions or
disagreements to completion or resolution; Don't talk openly or
directly about shameful, abusive, or compulsive behavior. In deed, it
was therapeutic for Stanley to admit he was molested. Admission of
the incident was part of his first step towards recovery that prepared
him to break the unspoken rules, accept the situation as exactly what
it was and gave him the opportunity to begin healing. An alcoholic
physician wrote in the book *Alcoholic Anonymous*: "And acceptance
is the answer to all my problems today. When I am disturbed, it is
because I find some person, place, thing, or situation – some fact of
life – unacceptable to me, and I can find no serenity until I accept that
person, place, thing, or situation as being exactly the way it is
supposed to be at this moment. Nothing, absolutely nothing, happens
in God's world by mistake. Until I could accept life completely on
life's term, I cannot be happy. I need to concentrate not so much on
what needs to be changed in the world as on what needs to be
changed in me and in my attitude."

Stanley's Story Continued

Admission of molestation was necessary for Stanley to begin his
journey into accepting his situation for what it is. When Stanley
returned for his next session, he was asked to explain in detail his first
encounter with his stepfather. He cried as though he had just gone
through the ordeal all over again. But that was not all. He was asked
to narrate exactly what happened the second time around, and then
third time, etc. As he neared the end of the narration, he cried less
and he looked exhausted. Then he was asked why he did not seek
help from another significant adult, since mom did not believe him
after the first encounter. He said his stepfather had threatened to hurt
him, if he told anybody. He said he 'hated' his stepfather. Next, the
counselor wanted to know about the first time when Stanley stole his
mom's drink, what he felt how soon he did it again. Then, the
counselor asked Stanley about his first marijuana smoke, what he felt
and how it changed the relationship with mom and stepfather.
Stanley recalled that after he started smoking marijuana, he began
resisting his stepfather's abuse and staying out late at his next door

neighbor's house with his friends. He said marijuana made him feel care free and independent: "I felt like I did not have to listen to my mom or stepfather." Stanley said marijuana actually freed him from family abuse. The counselor allowed Stanley to share the strength and victory he received from smoking marijuana for a brief moment before changing the direction of the session. So, "What was the first trouble you got into after smoking marijuana," the counselor asked. What was the next trouble?; And the next one, etc, etc. Stanley confessed that even though he did well in school, academically, marijuana was responsible for his being kicked out of high school. Clearly, at this point, Stanley understood the classic definition of self-defeating behavior as was presented in chapter three. Stanley left the office with a clear picture of his presenting problem, its precursor, origin, development and potential end result, if not arrested. All of these were accomplished in four sessions of counseling. The counselor had succeeded in not only confronting Stanley's inconsistencies, but has been able to 'connect dots,' which has positioned Stanley to be able to rethink on his convictions about the positive power of marijuana. The next phase in the treatment process was to determine how to help Stanley change his values, which will enable him to change his attitude and ultimately, his behavior.

Prochaska et al., (1992) indicated that individuals go through five stages of change when overcoming addictions, or changing other problem behaviors. Three of the stages precede the action stage, which is when people begin to take decisive behavioral steps to overcome their problems. These preliminary stages are called pre-contemplation (not thinking they have a problem or not admitting to one); at the contemplation (reflecting upon the possibility of having a problem, and on what to do about it) stage the client begins to recognize some consequences associated with addiction and begins to consider whether a change is necessary; the preparation (getting ready to take action) for change stage is characterized by the client considering various strategies to make changes in her/his substance use; in the action (doing something about the problem) stage the client begins to make the changes as planned; and in the change maintenance (staying in balance) stage, strategies are developed to maintain the gains. Many youths entering drug treatment would initially fall in the first two stages of change. It would be premature and inappropriate to teach them how to be drug-free. It would be far more timely and appropriate to engage them in a thought-provoking discussion about their drug use, trying to raise their consciousness. When youths are pressured to give up their drug using habit, they tend to resist and this destroys the necessary therapeutic alliance needed to implement change. Miller and Rollnick (1991) explained the resistance of drug abusing clients of all ages in terms of the psychological concept of ambivalence, which means simultaneously experiencing two different and opposing feelings and attitudes about something. Most drug-abusing youths are ambivalent about their drug use. They feel internal conflict. On the one hand, they see that they derive certain benefits from it. On the other hand, they also see potential harm. The nature of ambivalence is to maintain balance. If youths are pressured too much towards abstinence, they are likely to bounce back to drug use and if their drug use pushes them too far into rock bottom, they want treatment or some form of control over their drug use.

An alternate model to the stages of change is the Motivational Enhancement Therapy (MET) or simply Motivational Interviewing (MI). William Miller and colleagues (1991, 1992, 1995, 2000) developed this model. MI draws from Prochaska's "stages of change." Traditionally, substance abuse treatment programs (especially social model programs) see clients as either ready or not ready for treatment. This dichotomous perspective that clients are either ready or not ready for treatment underscores the fine gray between the two extremes. On the other hand, MI perspective sees clients as transitioning through several different stages of readiness to changes. The goal is to help clients move along the continuum from pre-contemplation towards action. This can be accomplished by using some of the techniques mentioned earlier: reflective listening, empathy, affirmation, probing with open-ended questions, etc. Shaffer and Robbins (1995) suggest that the counselor concentrate on exploration of the client's motivation to use substances as well as her/his reasons to stop or change. We referred to this earlier as the examination of ambivalence, which is the key to helping clients move along the stage of change continuum from the pre-contemplation stage into the contemplation stage, and ultimately toward the action stage. Shaffer and Robbins contend that it is ambivalence, not denial, that is the core issue in addiction treatment. The client invariably presents an internal struggle pulling them toward use of substances and simultaneously pulling them toward sobriety. The counselor, using skills and care, directs the client to understand how the use of substances conflict with the client's values. Providing objective, non-judgmental feedback about the consequences of the client's substance use, effects this technique. The motivation to change must come from the client. The counselor merely prods and facilitates a warm milieu for the client to become motivated to change through answering open-ended questions and examination of the advantages of making change. As the ambivalence is tipped in favor of a desire to make changes, the counselor uses other directive or strategic interventions to help the client proceed into the preparation for change and action stages. On a final note, it is important for the counselor to avoid prescribing a pre-determined method of achieving the identified goals. However, it can be helpful for the counselor to give the client advice on how to achieve goals if the client asks for it or the counselor checks with the client to find out whether she/he is interested in suggestions.

High impact aerobic exercise is a very effective primer of change when working with youths. They usually need a little motivation to begin the process, since they have no clue what its intended purpose is at the beginning. Each youth in the Job Corps treatment program is given the sample handout below and the succeeding 90-day workout plan, which is also used in the drug prevention education group. The handout teaches the youths about the importance of proper diet and exercise, while the actual physical aspect of exercise is taught in the gymnasium. Youths are generally reluctant to begin the exercise program, but once they begin, the first benefit is improved sleep due to increased detoxification of the drugs in their system on arrival to treatment. It is recommended that the exercise regimen begin as soon as drug test results are made available. One major symptom of marijuana detoxification is disrupted sleep. As with all drugs, the withdrawal symptoms are the exact opposite of the drug effect. Since marijuana relaxes the user to a point of sedation, it will have the opposite effect when usage is abruptly stopped. Another benefit of high impact exercise during early treatment for youths is the release of endorphins. When released in the brain cells endorphins causes a mild euphoric effect in youths, which allows the youths to recapture some of the feeling they crave in drug use. Exercise also relaxes the youths, especially those that have serious anger issue, and those that suffer anxiety as a result of detoxification of marijuana. Although all exercise at this stage of treatment is useful, one type of exercise is particularly recommended – aerobic weight lifting. Aerobic weight lifting is a structured weight lifting, which requires using multiple weight training equipments to target a specific muscle group. It requires youths to vigorously move from one equipment to another and do ten repetitions during each set for a minimum of three sets before taking a one-minute rest. A total of ten sets of ten repetitions are performed before using another set of equipments that target a different muscle group. This particular routine keeps the heart rate at optimum function for about 90 minutes. The intensity of the exercise forces the brain to release, among other chemicals, dopamine, norepinephrine, and serotonin. Youths are electrified, following a work out routine. Over a period of five weeks doing the exercise regimen for at least four times each week, youths begin to crave the after-effect of the intense exercise. Male youths will notice significant muscle development in ninety days, while female youths notice significant body sculpting as excess body fat is replaced with lean muscles.

HEALTH AND FITNESS:
A Healthy Goal For Sobriety
By Dr. Kay Wachuku

Health – Soundness, especially of body or mind. It is a condition of optimal well-being. Yoga teachings contend that one cannot house a healthy mind in an unhealthy body.
Fitness – A state of physical soundness: healthy.

The Four Basic Food Groups

The body needs food for nourishment. There are four basic food groups and other trace elements like minerals (calcium, sodium, magnesium, phosphorus, potassium, etc) that the body needs for nourishment.

<u>**Protein:**</u>
This is the body's building block for growing, maintaining, and repairing worn out cells. Without protein, our bodies could not regulate fluids and our immune systems would shut down. Protein produces hormones and enzymes. It is second only to water. When protein is eaten, the body breaks it down through a complex process called digestion. The final product is called amino acid. There are different stains of amino acid – L-Cartinine, L-Arginine, L-Lycine, etc. As with anything else, too much protein is not good. Excess protein is converted to fat and waste. Most of all, breaking down more protein than needed puts undue stress on the kidney. Moderate active, healthy adults need 45-65 grams of protein daily. Simply divide your body weight by 3 to find out approximately how much you need daily. It is important to note that protein breaks down slower than carbohydrate. This means that if you are dieting, eating more protein will curb your appetite longer than eating carbohydrate. Foods with protein include meat, fish, milk, egg, vegetables, nuts, etc. Too much animal protein raises serum cholesterol when compared to vegetable protein.

Carbohydrates (carb):

Carb supply the efficient fuel the body needs to function. It is the main source of the body's energy reserve. When eaten, the body breaks down carb into complex sugar – glucose and glycerol. It is stored in the muscles as glycogen and the rest is distributed in the body as adipose tissue. One of the liver's primary functions is to synthesize carb into sugar. Carb taken during prolonged exercise help boost endurance and delay fatigue, and helps alter brain neurotransmitter activities, which may, in turn, impact motor skill performance, mood and cognition. When the body does not have enough, it scavenges muscle for fuel. This leads to ketosis, a toxic condition resulting from disrupted metabolism. Excess carb stores as adipose tissue. There are two types of carb: simple and complex carb. Complex carb is the one we need. It comes from grains, fruits, nuts, potatoes, rice etc. Simple carb is refined or processed carb, such as white flour, sugar, pastries, etc. Simple carb burns too quickly and easily breakdown to poly-saturated fat. Simple carb is your regular 87 gas, while complex carb is your high octane 91 gas.

Fat:

Fat consists of the mono and poly-saturated types. It contains more calories than carb. It breaks down in the body to fatty acids and glycerol. It is also high in high-density cholesterol. The Surgeon General's Report warns that over consumption of dietary fat is a menace to the health of the American people. It ranks 5 of the top 10 leading causes of death in the United States. Heart disease, cancer, stroke, diabetes and arteriosclerosis are associated with dietary fat excesses or imbalance. Fat is an important nutrient that needs to be limited in our diet in other to reduce the risk of chronic disease.

Vitamins:

Vitamins are organic complex compounds essential for health. The body needs vitamins and minerals to grow, produce energy, fight disease, repair injured tissue and maintain normal health. Only tiny amounts of vitamins are required in the diet. Vitamins D, E, A, and K are fat soluble, while B12, biotin, B6, folic acid, C, niacin, thiamin, riboflavin are water-soluble. Problem arises if the body does not receive enough vitamins. For example, shortage of vitamin D = rickets, E = nerve damage, K = spontaneous bleeding, Foliate = anemia, C = scurvy, Niacin = pellagra, etc. *Food provides more than 20-plus vitamins and vegetables give an edge, as long as your nutrients are from the kitchen instead of the medicine cabinet.* Sources of vitamins are green foliate vegetables, fruits, meat, poultry, fish, eggs, grains, nuts, seeds, and dairy products.

Essential or Trace Elements:

These are inorganic compounds needed to maintain homeostasis. Examples are potassium, calcium, sodium, nitrogen, phosphorus, etc. They are also found in food. Others are food additives like cooking salt.

EXERCISE AND FITNESS

Exercise is any activity requiring physical exertion done for the sake of health. Activities range from walking and yoga to lifting weights and martial arts. Regular exercise as a way of promoting health can be traced back at least 5,000 years to India, where yoga originated. In China, exercise involving martial arts, such as t'ai chi, kung fu, developed possibly 2,500 years ago. The ancient Greek had exercise programs, which led to the first Olympic games in 726 B.C. Only within the last 100 years have the medical and scientific communities documented the benefits that even light but regular exercise has on physical and mental health.

Benefits of Exercise:

The medical community recognizes that regular exercise, along with a proper diet, is one of the two most important factors in maintaining good physical and mental health, and preventing and managing many diseases. One study of 13,000 people followed for 8 years showed that people who walk 30 minutes a day have a significantly reduced risk of premature death than people who did not exercise regularly. Walking and other cardiovascular exercise can reduce the risk of heart disease, some cancer, hypertension, arthritis, osteoporosis, stroke, and depression. More recently, it has become clear that exercise may be a therapeutic tool in a variety of patients with or at risk for diabetes.

BODY SCULPTING AND WEIGHT CONTROL THROUGH WEIGHT LIFTING

Adding weight lifting to your fitness repertoire not only builds muscles and boosts endurance, but it can help lose weight and get you in shape faster than walking or jogging alone. This is because muscles use more calories than fat, even when at rest. The more muscle the body has, the more calories it burns. Burned calories equal burned pounds. Studies have shown that working out twice a week is 90% as effective for building strength and muscle size as working out three days a week. I recommend three days a week for youths. It assures you will attain that hard body you've always wanted 10% faster. Weight training not only tones your muscles, but it also raises your basal metabolism, which causes you to burn more calories. In addition to burning extra calories without even trying, weight training also reduces the risk of osteoporosis, and the development of adult-onset diabetes. Weight training reduces fat, speeds metabolism, increases endurance, improves posture, strengthens bones and cuts risk of injury.

Benefits Cross Age/Gender Lines:
*Tufts University, Medford, MA, put a group of elderly nursing home residents on a weight lifting regimen. They all more than doubled their strengths. Four people traded in their walkers for canes in 10 weeks.

*In another Tuft study, a group of post-menopausal women performed twice-weekly weight training at levels comparable to women 15-20 years younger. They pumped up their muscle power 35% to 76% and as a result, burned 442 more calories each week while at rest.

*A Brigham Young University study found that 30 women who did nine basic weight training exercise three times a week for 12

96

weeks cut their daily fat intake to 30% of total calories. The control group of women that stretched instead of weight lifting made no improvements, according to the Journal of American Dietetic Association.

Muscle lost to aging can be replaced by weight lifting, says Wayne Wescott, strength consultant to the national YMCA. Each decade, the average American man loses about 7 pounds of muscle and the average woman about 5 pounds of muscle. Studies show that two to three months of strength training can replace three pounds of muscle. By lifting weights, you counter your body's natural metabolic decline of 2 to 5% each decade. That's why it is vital to weight loss, says James M. Rippe, M.D., author of fit over forty. The American Heart Association (AHA) says pumping iron is also good for the heart. The AHA says that for healthy adults, and some cardiac patients, a regular program of weight training not only increases muscle strength and endurance, it also improves function of the heart and lungs, enhances glucose metabolism, reduces coronary disease risk factors and boosts well-being. "After reviewing the literature, we came to the rather startling conclusion that resistance training, like aerobic exercise, can improve cardiovascular function and favorably modify many of the risk factors associated with coronary heart disease," says physiologist Barry A. Franklin, Director of cardiac rehabilitation program at William Beaumont Hospital in Royal Oak, Michigan.

DIET: THE FINAL FRONTIER

When it comes to weight loss, fitness and exercise, diet plays a significant role in fitness goal attainment. Eating a healthy diet that is low in fat and sugar, and high in fiber, can cut the risk of heart disease, cancer, diabetes, stroke, and osteoporosis. A good diet must include all four basic food groups. Skipping meals is not a good diet plan. Nor is drinking your meal good.

HINT FOR BEGINNING YOUR WEIGHT PROGRAM
* Do what you enjoy

* Learn the proper technique
* Start slow and low
* Engage all the muscles
* Rest

Should I Take Weight Training Supplements?

Yes. No. Yes, if you do not eat right or if you eat mostly junk food. No, if you use the above information to formulate a healthy diet plan that includes proper rest. Don' forget to eat lots of fruits and nut for vitamins.

REFERENCES

Journal of the American Dietetic Association
Surgeon General's 1977 Report
Journal of American Medical Association
Fit Over Forty by James M. Rippe
American Heart Association 1998 publication
Backwoods Home Magazine, May-June 2002 issue
JETonline May 28, 2001 issue
Gale Encyclopedia of Medicine
Nutrition Today, July-August, 1998

90-Day High Impact, Body Priming/Weight Training Program

MON	LEGS 30-40 min	BACK 30-40 min	ABS 15 - 20 min
	*Leg raises - 5sets of 25 reps *Squats - 10 sets of 10 reps (pyramid) *Leg presses - 5 sets of 10 reps	*Dead lifts - 10 sets of 10 reps *Pull downs - 5 sets of 10 reps *Standing bent over rows - 5 sets of 10 reps	*Decline sit ups - 10 sets of 12 reps *Crunches - 5 sets of 10 reps Ab rollers - 10 sets of 10 reps
TUE	CHEST 30 -40 min.	SHOULDERS 30 - 40 min	ABS 15 TO 20 min
	*Flat bench - 10 sets of 10 reps (pyramid) *Incline - 5 sets of 10 reps *Decline - 5 sets of 10 reps	*Military presses - 10 sets of 10 reps (pyramid) *Dumb bell flies - 5 sets of 10 reps *Dumb bell presses - 5 sets of 10 reps	*Leg raises - 10 sets of ten reps *Cable crunches - 5 sets of 12 reps *Sit ups - 5 sets of 10 reps
THU	BICEPS - 30 - 40 min	TRICEPS - 30 to 40 min	ABS 15 to 20 min
	*Curls 10 sets of 10 reps (pyramid) *Dumb bell concentration curls - 5 sets of 10 reps *Preacher bench curls - 5 sets of 10 reps	*Skull crushers - 10 sets of 10 reps (pyramid) *Standing French presses - 5 sets of 10 reps *Cable pull downs 5 sets of 10 reps	*Flat bench crunches seven sets of 25 reps *Ab rollers 5 sets of 10 reps *Sit ups - 5 sets of 10 reps

FRI	LEGS/CHEST 30 - 40 min	LATS/BACK/SHOULDER 30 - 40 min	ABS 15 - 20 min
	*Seated calve raises 5 sets of 20 reps *Hack squats 5 sets of reps *Dumb bell flat bench presses 5 sets of 10 reps *Dumb bell incline/decline presses 5 sets of 10 reps	*Cable pull downs 5 sets of 10 reps *Dumb bell "lawn mowers" 5 sets of 10 reps *Seated cable lat pulls 5 sets of 10 reps *Military presses 5 sets of 10 reps	*Leg raises 10 sets of 10 reps * Seated crunches 5 sets of 10 reps *Decline sit ups 10 sets of 10 reps.

P/s, rest for 15 seconds between sets and 2 minutes between body parts. Drink lots of water. Rest on Wednesday, Saturday and Sunday. Expect your body to be very sore due to the high repetition. Avoid fried food. Cut back on your carbohydrate and sugar intake. Eat lots of lean meat and vegetables. GOOD LUCK!!!

In fact, aerobic weight lifting is very highly therapeutic when used in conjunction with counseling and prevention education. It increased retention in the treatment program and drastically reduced relapse by about 75% in the award-winning Inland Empire Job Corps Center youth program.

Let's return back to Stanley. He had been in treatment for about five weeks. During this period, he had learned to use exercise to relax, undergone catharsis, learned that his use of marijuana and alcohol was somehow a coping strategy for his physical and emotional abuse, seen the connection between marijuana use and dropping out of high school, learned to experience euphoria through exercise, and most of all, has experienced sobriety for five weeks. He had detoxified well enough to overcome the initial symptoms of marijuana detoxification: headache, sleeplessness, anxiety, lack of appetite, irritability, mild paranoia, etc. In fact, he was beginning to feel good about himself, even though he experiences sporadic bouts of the urge to use marijuana every so often. To add to his advantage, he had received some monetary allowance from the Job Corps program, which he had used to buy himself some decent clothing. There appears to be a glimpse of hope returning to Stanley, yet there was the general suspicion, based on ambivalence that somehow, all of this might be a set up for him to fail. This is the stage in Stanley's treatment that calls for another unorthodox counseling technique for working with youths. This technique is called the "Retroactive" approach. It uses "Retropolation" to explore Stanley's motivation for change, and to lure Stanley away from the negative end of his ambivalence. Retropolation requires that the counselor take Stanley back on a total recall of the worst of his experiences during his drug use days. It mimics the abreaction technique, but instead of igniting catharsis, Stanley is goaded through vivid imagery of the negative aspects of his drug use adventure days, with a view to exploring potential outcome, should he have remained on the continuum of drug abuse adventure. The exercise calls for a conclusion. In other words, Stanley is directed to play the imaginary tape of his drug use experience through to the end, making sure that each negative detailed is highlighted along the continuum. Often, conclusions such as going to jail, being institutionalized, or even death are reached. Once these conclusions are reached, the counselor then skillfully turns the imagery around. This time the counselor tries to create value 'here and now.' Using a similar, but antithetical approach to Retropolation, the counselor guides to Stanley explore the positive end of the ambivalence – Post Recovery Approach. Stanley is asked to imagine not using drugs for a year. He is directed to envision himself completing his vocational training, getting a good paying job, getting his own affordable apartment, buying his own somewhat of a used car, having the opportunity to invite his younger brother to come visit him in his apartment, and saving lots of money, since he will no longer spend money on drugs. The end result is usually value created on the 'here and now' and hope buttressed to a point of craving this imaginary, yet attainable goal. What this approach does, in effect, is to pick Stanley up and leave him in fear of falling. Remember our proverbial African philosophy that he who is down need not fear falling. Well, now Stanley is up and will fear falling. He suddenly realizes that he has something to loose, should he go back to the old ways of doing things. This positive type of fear is the foundation on which most successful ventures are built. Retropolation is a very powerful tool in working with youths and adults who are resistant to treatment – adults who consider themselves 'chronic relapsers.' From a feelings analysis, Retropolation stirs up feelings of hopelessness, fear and sadness. It usually leaves the client exhausted at the end of the exercise. By contrast, Post Recovery Approach stirs up hope, willingness to change and quest for a happy ending. The client feels elated and ready to begin the journey of recovery.

GROUP COUNSELING FOR YOUTHS: HOW IT WORKS

Behavioral therapy offers a wide range of different treatment methods. Individual counseling is effective in attempting to examine and make changes to maladaptive behavior. However, some clients and observers tend to perceive the counselor as artificially molding the clients' problems to suite the counselor's own preconceived theoretical notions of what an acceptable behavior should be. Group therapy offers a solution to this suspect situation in therapy. The group experience is a complementary workshop experience to the individual analysis; each is enriched by the other. In group therapy, a small group of clients (usually no more than twelve) meet regularly to discuss their problems, while the counselor moderates and directs the flow of the group discussion. Inherent in the group process is the enhancing of the experiential dimension. Instead of trying to pry underlying issues out of a client in individual counseling, the issues are lived and felt in group counseling. Something that may have been thrashed around for weeks in individual sessions becomes suddenly a gut experience in the group. Issues come to the fore that would be unlikely to arise in individual sessions. Group counseling attempts to give individuals a safe and comfortable place where they can work out problems and emotional issues. Clients gain insight into their own thoughts and behavior, and offer suggestions and support to others. In addition, clients who have a difficult time with interpersonal relationships can benefit from the social interactions that are a basic part of the group counseling experience. Several techniques may be deployed in group therapy. For example, Psychodrama, Gestalt techniques, sensitivity training, and ritualizations may be employed. The counselor may be more active in group sessions than she/he could allow in individual sessions, and the transference to the counselor is lessoned considerably. The counselor may be responded to more like the human being she/he is rather than the archetypal role thrust upon him or her in individual analysis. Often this permits negative attitudes to surface in the group, attitudes that the counselor would have been too frightened to raise in individual counseling.

The selection of the group is usually based on what the clients might gain from or offer to the group interaction. The group may homogeneous or heterogeneous, depending on whether members have similar diagnostic background or different emotional issues. Group membership may be open or closed to new members once the group is formed. Some counselors prefer a closed group, so as to prevent disruption of the group bonding process. Others allow new group members to come with careful screening and indoctrination. The number of sessions varies, depending on the makeup, goals, and type of group. For example, a hospital inpatient group may last six weeks, whereas, a social model in-house group may last up to six to eighteen months. The prime goal of group therapy is self-discovery. Depending on the goal of the group and the training of the counselor, the group may take its own direction or the counselor may direct the flow of interaction. Often the counselor does some of both, providing direction when the group gets off track while letting them set their own agenda. The counselor may guide the group by simply reinforcing the positive behaviors they engage in. For example, if a group member shows empathy to another member, or offer a constructive suggestion, the counselor will point this out and explain the value of these actions to the group. In almost all group therapy situations, the counselor will attempt to emphasize the common traits among group members so that members can gain a sense of group identity. It allows group members to realize that others face the same issues they do. The main benefit group therapy may have over individual counseling is that some clients behave and react more like themselves in a group setting than they would in individual counseling. The group therapy clients gain a certain sense of identity and social acceptance from their membership in the group; they are surrounded by other members who share the same anxieties and emotional issues that the individual clients have. Seeing how others deal with these issues may give them new solutions to their problems. Feedback from group members also offers them a unique insight into their own behavior, and the group provides a safe forum in which to practice new behaviors. Further, by helping others in group work through their problems, group therapy members can gain more self-esteem. Group experience may also simulate family experiences of clients and will allow family dynamics issues to emerge. It is important to note that not all clients will benefit from group therapy. Clients who display grossly bizarre or inappropriate behavior, delusions, thought disorders, and other signs of 'psychosis' should be referred to a psychiatrist or a psychiatric facility. Similarly, evidence of strong homicidal or suicidal tendencies often requires medical and custodial intervention. Despite all the advantages of group therapy, care must be exercised during the initial intake into the group not to create an aversive-aversive conflict for the new group member. This is especially note worthy when working with youths. We contended earlier that youths want to be in control. They despise the idea of someone else or some small group controlling their lives. Many youths have left treatment because of the so-called aversion-aversion conflict – a situation in which the individual finds her/himself equally repelled by two alternative courses of action. For example, a youth who came to treatment because she/he realized that drug use has taken control over her/his free will or causing her/him too much negative consequence (avoidance response) may find treatment equally repelling, if she/he thinks the treatment group is exerting the same control she/he is trying to avoid. Remember that drug-abusing youths suffer terminal uniqueness and want to be in control.

GIBSON HOUSE EXPERIENCE

Many years ago the author had the opportunity to work with a local in-house social model treatment center, Gibson House for Men. The program is one of the most successful centers in the area.

Majority of the clients who left the program did so within the first 48 hours of arrival. Many of those clients who left were youths. At the time in question, treatment outcome and state grant accountability were not hot issues, so programs did not spent much time on treatment outcome research. In retrospect, it is clear the reason some of those youths left was as a result of aversion-aversion conflict. The Gibson House program was very confrontational. Clients were broken down to submit to being addicted and virtually humiliated in other to qualify for treatment. The in-house group made the ultimate decision as to whether a client is admitted into the program or not. The in-take process was very rigorous. First a prospective client calls; he is told there is no bed available, even if in reality there is bed. The client is then instructed to call daily until a bed is available. A prospective client must make the calls in other to be admitted into the program. Calls by another individual or agency on behalf of the client are not acceptable. The reasoning is that the prospective client has to show some level of willingness to enter the program. After two or more calls, the prospective client is asked how far she/he lives from the program site. She/he is then instructed to arrive at a predetermined time, usually within an hour of calling, depending on the distance from the program. Failure to make the deadline was grounds for disqualification. Once again, the logic is that the prospective client has to show seriousness about joining the program.

Finally, the prospective client arrives. One of the counselors, who usually was a graduate from the program with no formal training in counseling other than the tradition of treatment handed down to the counselor by the counselor's predecessors, hands the prospective client a treatment contract. A brief psych-social assessment is done to determine the prospective clients drugs of choice. The prospective client is then ready for a massive 'shock and awe' eligibility for admission exercise. On the average, the treatment center has about 30 to 40 resident clients on any given day. Thirty to forty chairs are lined up in two parallel lines facing each other. At the end of the two rows of chairs is one empty chair standing aside, but between the two rows of chair. Resident clients are seated in the two rows of parallel chairs facing each other with just enough space between the two rows for a person to walk through. The prospective client is brought in by the in-take counselor and seated in the lonely, empty chair to the far end of the two parallel rows of chair, away from everybody. The prospective client is then ready for the 'first encounter of the worst kind.' The first question is usually: "What do you love most in life?" The unsuspecting prospective client will usually give any one of the following answers – my wife, mom, dad, children, grandmother/father, girl/boy friend, to mention but a few. Once the answer is given, the group of 30 to 40 men yell loader than thunder in unison: "Bullsh-t." The prospective client is then told that he loved his drug or alcohol more than whatever answer she/he gave. Again, the prospective client is asked: "Have you ever stolen form someone." Once again, the innocent unsuspecting prospective client answers honestly – no. "Bullsh-t," the group resounds. The prospective client is then told that all the money spent on drugs or alcohol was money stolen from loved ones. Here is the funny question: "Are you suicidal or homicidal?" The prospective client honestly says no, and you know the routine by now. The prospective client is told that using drugs or alcohol was an act of installmental suicide and that if the prospective client has ever offered any one else drugs or alcohol, it was an act of installmental homicide. Many prospective clients are in tears within twenty minutes of this torturous confrontation. Those that do not show any emotion are denied entrance into the group. If the prospective client breaks down in tears, additional drilling questions are initiated. The prospective client is confronted in every phase of her/his possible denial mechanism until the prospective client accedes to being addicted or ready to make a change. A few prospective clients will leave before the process is over. Many will be in shock for about twenty-four hours before motioning to leave. Once the group admits a prospective client and the client expresses intention to leave the group, a special session is assembled. This session usually deploys scare tactics for retention. The client is reminded that

"Brother Ass" (nickname for addiction) is outside the door waiting to devour the client. The client is told that in the last twenty-four hours, while the group is trying to save her/him, "Brother Ass" was outside doing pushups, waiting to knock the client down again. Upon successful admission into the group, the client is faced with the same intensity of attack in group therapy. Clients are psychologically coerced to admit and confess to events that they may not have actually experienced, just to satisfy the group expectation. In time the client is brain washed into 'group think' – A situation in which the client begins to think like everyone else in the group, almost devoid of her/his own independent thinking in matters of personal importance. The client is asked to bring all personal matters of importance to the group for consideration and approval by the group before any action is taken. Those who do not accept group recommendation are accused of acting on self-will or not acting in 'principle.' Failure to comply with group recommendation will often times lead to a vote to get the client out of the group. In the case of a less severe disobedience to group suggestion or recommendation, group members are asked to make a sacrifice on behalf of the client who refused to take group advise. Sometimes the disobedient group member is humiliated by asking her/him to wear a sign that reads: "I will obey my group members' orders" for one week. In retrospect, there is no doubt that many youths who usually are terminally unique or want control will suffer aversion-aversion conflict when confronted with the Gibson House treatment modality. These youths will repel the consequences of their drug use as much as they will repel the alternative course of action – the Gibson House for Men 'shock and awe' treatment protocol. This, in turn, will lead to treatment failure. Over the years, the Gibson House for Men treatment program has softened up on the attack therapy. As county and federal grantors demand accountability and treatment outcome reports, many social model treatments have modified their treatment protocol.

J.C. MODEL

As was noted earlier youths generally prefer individual counseling, because it is less invasive than group therapy. Many youths do not feel comfortable discussing their problems or their family problems in group setting. With that in mind, the Inland Empire Job Corps (J.C.) youth treatment program was designed to lessen anxiety among youths. The group is open entry/open exit. That means, newly recruited clients may enter the group, while those that have completed their five months mandated treatment might proceed to after care groups. Group therapy begins as a mild sharing session. The counselor begins the group with educational information targeted at eliciting information from youths. For example, the counselor begins the session by saying that many youths do not use drugs because: they have low self-esteem, were raised in bad neighborhood, are stupid or because their parents use drugs. Nor, do youths use drugs purely because of peer pressure, The counselor then asserts that youths generally use drugs because it fun to use drugs. At this point the youths are roused up in excitement to hear their notion confirmed by their counselor. This type of introduction often primes the youth to discuss the issue further. However, the skilled counselor takes the discussion off to another tangent. The counselor adds that with most youths, drug use helps sooth some emotional injuries sustained in early childhood, such as abuse from a stepparent, incest, or even favoritism towards a brother/sister, etc. The counselor stops and goes back to his earlier contention that many youths use drugs because it is fun. The counselor then asks for feedback on the topic. At this point almost every youth in the group is eager to speak. Some are even allowed to romanticize their old drug use fantasies. Many traditional substance abuse counselors will not tolerate this type of discussion in group. However, under the J.C. model this type of discussion is craftily used to get to the more serious issues. The idea is to get youths to begin to talk freely.

Once they are able to talk freely, the counselor then directs the discussion to a therapeutic level. Some group members who came into the program denying ever using drugs, usually find themselves admitting trying drug use once or twice during this initial discussion. Others remain in denial for a longer period before acceding to drug use. The counselor is very alert during this somewhat of permissive discussion. Any discussion that falls under dangerous grounds – suicide, harm to others, homicide, or rape is immediately dealt with in appropriate manner. Once group members are comfortable with the discussion, the counselor skillfully reverts the discussion to emotional injury. Usually, there is always that one youth who gets 'carried away' and proceeds to talk about how his stepfather molested him. The counselor quickly points out that it was not the youth's fault that such a terrible thing happened. The counselor then asks the group to not be judgmental, but to take three minutes of silence to think about what they just heard before the discussion continues. During this moment of silence, some youths may start showing emotions they never knew they had. In fact, some have been known to start crying. Suddenly the domino effect begins. Of course, there is always "Mr. Hardcore" who is too strong to show emotion. We do not worry about him because we know his day is coming. After the moment of silence, the group is asked to examine what happened to see if it could have happened to anybody, given the same circumstance. The counselor tries to emphasize the fact that there are bad people in life who will take advantage of opportunity to project their wrong doing on others. From this point on, other issues begin to surface, buttressing the session with nothing but abreaction/catharsis. Everybody is given a fair chance to participate. Those who do not participate are not chastised, harassed, nor reprimanded. Instead the counselor simply says: "maybe Andrew has never experienced any of these things. We should not make him lie." The counselor knows fully well that eventually Andrew will talk. This non-judgmental and permissive gesture towards denial actually helps youths prepare to table their issues when time permits. The counselor unwinds the session by acknowledging those who have ventured to face their issues head-on and assures those who participated that hope and recovery is unfolding.

James' Story

James was the youth who tested positive for marijuana (1020ng/ml) on entry into the J.C. program. He denied he nor anyone in his family has ever used drugs. As usual, he was told he would have to go through the motion of being in treatment for six months, although his test result may have been erroneous. It was standard practice to allow youths to deny drug use and yet include them in treatment. During individual counseling, James was told that his sessions would consist of drug prevention education – something anyone would benefit from. He was however, told that he will have to participate in group therapy the best he can, till his time is served. In group therapy James introduced himself and boldly announced that he has never used drugs. One client immediate interrupted: "Denial is not a River in Egypt." The TEAP counselor cautioned: "Be nice guys. Some people are here because of different reasons, so let's not make fun of anybody." For the next three months, James participated in group therapy holding his denial grounds. During one of the opening sessions when past drug use was being glamorized, James almost slipped. He said he knows that drug use could be fun. A group member quickly challenged him and asked how he could possibly know that, since he had never used drugs before. James responded that he has observed one of his cousins smoke marijuana a few times and that his cousin seems to be having fun whenever he used that 'stuff.' So, James continued with his denial. In fact, he often said he was lucky to have ended up in a group with a bunch of marijuana smokers. He said he was learning enough information that would allow him to help his cousin stop his marijuana habit. During the third month of group participation James was finally confronted in a very subtle manner. The group was discussing how healthy families resolve issues and build resiliency into children to keep them from using drugs. James was asked to share with the group how his family was able to raise him to say no to drugs. James stared by saying that his father always warned that if he ever saw him (James) use drugs, he would peel his butt off. He said his mom's strategy was to buy him and his brother nice things, so that way they did not have to use drugs. James was then asked to think of a childhood serious problem he had and share with the group how his family helped him go through it. The group was asked to give James three minutes of silence to allow him to think deep. After about two minutes of silence, James said: "My name is James. I guess I have to stop bulls—ting you guys. I am an addict too." Surprisingly, the group gave him a standing ovation and began chanting 'welcome, welcome, welcome.' Then the chanting stopped. James began to pour his soul out. All the hurt and emotion he had held on to for so long began to flow out of him. At some point he said he could not take it anymore. He began crying. The group was asked to show him some love. Everybody got up and gave him a peace hug. It takes what it takes for some people. All the group has to do is show compassion, and tolerance.

Society tends to focus on the physiological damage associated with drug use. As a result, preventive measures carry messages that are sometimes incongruent to the most damage sustained from drug use. The early 1990s saw a television commercial that shows an egg on a hot grill. The commercial then suggests that that is what happens to the brain when drugs are used. Well, many young people and adults who have ever used drugs quickly dismissed the claim as a gross exaggeration and thereby downplayed the real danger associated with drug use and abuse. The worst damage society suffers from drug abuse is not physiological. The subtle, but persistent and progressive destructive pattern of behavior associated with drug use poses more challenge to humanity than physiological damage. Medical science has made remarkable advances in treating physiological injuries, but psychological and emotional injuries are still a challenge to medical science. Drug abuse generally does more damage to the psych than it does to the physical body. In fact, marijuana does more mental damage to youths than it does to their physical body. Mental damage such as distorted thinking, amotivational syndrome, paranoia, depression, etc cost society a fortune. It is imperative that we seriously explore more new ways to help youths recover from mental illness associated with marijuana abuse. This book does not propose that the techniques explored in the preceding chapters are the only or best-known techniques for working with youths. There are other methods that have been proven effective. In recent times many substance abuse treatment professionals are beginning to come to a consensus that effective programs must use eclectic methods. Chapter six examines old and new ways of treatment that are equally effective.

CHAPTER SIX

THE ECLECTIC GRILL

Marijuana Impaired Youth is a book whose primary purpose is to highlight practical approaches in dealing with youths in treatment, while educating the general public about the subtle, serious psycho-neurophysiologic damage associated with marijuana abuse. The book does not claim to offer the only remedy to 'curing' youth drug abuse impairment. Nor, is the book a panacea for dealing with all youth drug abuse problems. The recommendation is that the counselor or therapist draws from a multi-model therapy in other to offer a wide array of effective treatment practices. This is probably the best approach, since most of our experiences comprise moving, feeling, sensing, imagining, thinking, and relating to one another. To that effect, we are bio-chemical-neurophysiologic entities. Our conduct is a product of ongoing behaviors, affective processes, sensations, images, cognitions, interpersonal relationships, and biological functions. A cognitive malfunction in youths, whether it is congenital, hereditary, or drug abuse induced, requires a systematic therapy that rests primarily on the theoretical base of social learning theory (Bandura, 1969, 1977, 1986) while also drawing from general system theory (Bertalanffy, 1974; Buckley, 1967) and group communication theory (Watzlawick, Weakland & Fisch, 1974). Combining these theories and other behavioral theories is the essence of effective clinical practice. In deed, it is the matrix of the "eclectic grill." For there seems to be no postulates or paradigms in these theoretical systems that are mutually contradictory or incompatible – they blend harmoniously into a congruent framework. This is what has been referred to as eclecticism: the selection and organization into a theoretical system of compatible findings or points of view, especially with a view to offering the best treatment protocol for dealing with substance abuse or other psychological abnormalities. Clinical effectiveness is predicated on the counselor's flexibility, versatility, and technical eclecticism. The theoretical eclectic tends to draw from diverse systems that may be epistemologically incompatible, whereas the technical eclectic uses procedures drawn from different sources without necessarily subscribing to the theories or disciplines that spawned them. The upshot is a consistent, systematic, and testable set of beliefs and assumptions about youths and their problems, and an armamentarium of effective therapeutic strategies for remedying drug induced impairment sustained by youths.

Eclecticism was not always welcomed in the substance abuse treatment field, simply because early success in alcoholism treatment was guided by a narrow view of the twelve-step program. Many counselors, who themselves were the final products of the twelve-step intervention, felt certain that long and lasting successful treatment for addiction can only be accomplished through the unilateral application of the twelve-step program. The first edition of the book *Alcoholics Anonymous* clearly advances this unilateral approach to recovery: "But there is One who has all power – that One is God. You must find Him now!" In later editions of the book the authors feared the implication of such a coercive command on agnostics and atheists and changed the last sentence to read: "May you find Him now." Of course, clinicians from schools of psychological thought have always advocated divergent methods of treatment, each strongly believing they have the best method. A close examination of the claims and counterclaims of the proponents of each school of thought reveals a number of trends or clusters. There are those who advocate particular techniques or procedures and tout them as virtual panaceas. Thus, one finds relaxation pundits, medication gurus, scream advocates, and promulgators of megavitamins, hypnosis, psychodrama, rebirthing, or some other unilateral intervention. These one-track procedures are the antithesis of eclectic therapy, which views human disquietude as multilayered and multileveled and calls for the correction of deviant behaviors, unpleasant feelings, negative sensations, intrusive images, irrational beliefs, stressful relationships, and physiological difficulties, through multidisciplinary application of all applicable schools of thought in dealing with one client's problem. The work of Arnold A. Lazarus was remarkable in advancing eclecticism in substance abuse treatment. In 1965 he wrote a paper on the need to treat alcoholism from a multidimensional perspective. The main components involved:

- Medical care to return the patient to physical well-being
- Aversion therapy and anxiety-relief conditioning to mitigate the patient's uncontrolled drinking
- A thorough assessment to identify "specific stimulus antecedents of anxiety" in the patient's environment
- The use of additional techniques, including systematic desensitization, assertiveness training, behavior rehearsal, and hypnosis
- The development of a cooperative relationship with the patient's spouse

Lazarus (1965) summarized all of the above in a statement: "the emphasis in psychological rehabilitation must be on a synthesis which would embrace a diverse range of effective therapeutic techniques, as well as innumerable adjunctive measures, to form part of a wide and all-embracing re-educative programme." Lazarus was suspicious of the effectiveness of what he called a narrow band behavior therapy, hence, he published "Broad-spectrum behavior Therapy and the Treatment of Agoraphobia" in 1966. His findings have become the basis for multimodal therapy, which has proven effective in treating many behavioral problems. This method of treatment now goes beyond the confines of private practices and has been applied in such diverse environments as mental hospitals, residential treatment facilities, out patient clinics, and complete care systems. Eclecticism is not merely a juxtaposition or conglomeration of psychoanalysis, behavior therapy, and many other systems. Instead, eclecticism calls for a careful assessment of a client's problem from a global perspective. It involves a thorough analysis of the client's presenting problem, non-conscious processes, defensive reactions to repressed emotional injuries, and projections, with a view to using theoretical base of social learning theory, general system theory, group and communication theory and technical eclecticism to formulate a treatment plan that addresses all facets of the client's problem. A Carl Rogers proponent may argue that his person-centered approach offers the therapist genuineness, empathy, and unpossessive caring to all clients, which is sufficient for therapeutic growth and change. On the contrary, fundamental to eclecticism is the emphasis that people have diverse needs and expectancies, come from very different molds, and require a wide range of stylistic, tactical, and strategic maneuvers from the counselor/therapist. Beside, no amount of empathy, genuineness, or unpossessive caring is likely to fill the gaps left by impoverished learning histories, behavioral and attitudinal deficits. These require teaching, coaching, training, modeling, shaping, and directing. These are measures that can only be attained through eclectic application. Lets examine some specific therapeutic applications, knowing that these applications may not solve all of a client's problems as a stand-alone therapy.

GESTALT APPROACH

In chapter five we learned that the psychological harm associated with drug abuse poses more danger to society than the physiologic harm. Psychological or emotional problems stymies economic productivity and hinder productive communication, which facilitates harmonious social living. Unfortunately, few medications are able to correct or remedy psychological problems. Even when medication is able to control excessive psychological disturbances in an individual, it falls short of teaching the individual subdued cognitive function. For this very reason, it is imperative that other measures are sort in other to harness fruitful resurgence from the psychological or emotionally dysfunctional individual. One such known effective measure is psychotherapy – a means of treating psychological or emotional problems such as neurosis or personality disorders through verbal and nonverbal communication. It is the treatment of psychological distress through talking with a specially trained therapist and learning new ways to cope rather than merely using medication to alleviate the distress. It is done with the immediate goal of aiding the psychologically sick person in increasing self-knowledge and awareness of relationships with others. Psychotherapy is carried out to assist people in becoming more conscious of their unconscious thoughts, feelings, and motives. The long-term goal of psychotherapy is making it possible for people to exchange destructive pattern of behavior for healthier, more successful ones.

Whenever psychotherapy is successful, humanity adds another productive and responsible individual to its assembly line. There are generally different approaches to psychotherapy, each believing strongly on its own merits to help clients resolve psychological problems. Three approaches, among others, are the most widely used: 1. The psychodynamic approach developed from the work of Austrian physician Sigmund Freud (1856-1939). Psychoanalytic therapeutic approach is founded on the notion that behavior and personality develop in relation to unconscious wishes and conflicts from childhood. 2. The behavioral approach encompasses various behavior modification techniques and theories, including assertiveness training/social skills training, operant conditioning, hypnosis/hypnotherapy, sex therapy, systematic desensitization, and others. 3. The cognitive approach stresses the role that thought plays in influencing behavior. Rational-emotive therapy and reality therapy are both examples of the cognitive approach. To the extent that each of these schools of psychological thoughts are effective, eclecticism dictates that they do not have to be mutually exclusive from each other. A client undergoing psychoanalytic therapy can also benefit from the social skills training that comes form behavioral approach. The client may also benefit from knowing that events in and of themselves do not upset people, but that people get upset about events because of their attitudes toward the events. In other words, using a cognitive approach can also help a psychoanalytic therapist and client reach their goals more effectively. This is the essence of the eclectic grill. Let us examine in detail the Gestalt therapy developed by Frederick (Fritz) Perls in the 1940s as a psychodynamic approach.

Gestalt therapy technique focuses on the events of the present, rather than in the past. A client's experience and behavior is approached holistically and not as independently functioning disparate parts. The underlying principle is that behavior must be studied in all its complexity rather than separated into discrete components, and that perception, learning, and other cognitive functions should be seen as structured wholes. Gestalt practitioners believed that mental experience was dependent not on a simple combination of elements but on the organization and patterning of experience and of one's perceptions. Thus they held that behavior must be studied in all its complexity rather than separated into discrete components, and that perception, learning, and other cognitive functions should be seen as structured wholes. The main aim of Gestalt approach is self-awareness. This is accomplished through exploration and resolution of interpersonal issues. The gestalt method teaches therapists and clients the phenomenological method of awareness, in which perceiving, feeling, and acting are distinguished from interpreting and reshuffling preexisting attitudes. Explanations and interpretations are considered less reliable than what is directly perceived and felt. The goal is for clients to become aware of what they are doing, how they are doing it, and how they can change themselves, and at the same time, to learn to accept and value themselves. The approach focuses more on process (what is happening) than content (what is being discussed). The emphasis is on what is being done, thought, and felt at the moment rather than on what was, might be, could be, or should be. Gestalt therapy is effective in individual, couples, and family therapies, as well as in therapy with children. We discussed the art of healing emotional injuries in chapter five. Gestalt lends itself to such healing, since it guides the client to identify current sensations, and emotions, particularly ones that are painful or disruptive. Clients are confronted with their unconscious feelings and needs, and are assisted to accept and assert those repressed parts of themselves. Gestalt therapy treats what is subjectively felt in the present, as well as what is objectively observed, as real and important in the healing process. This approach contrasts with approaches that treat what the client experiences as mere appearances and uses interpretation to find real meaning.

Chapter three examined the deadly harm that youths suffer when marijuana abuse alters their brain chemistry and causes them to adopt several forms of self-defeating behavior such as terminal uniqueness syndrome. In those altered states of mind, awareness of what is real is lost. This, in turn, leads to loss of insight, thereby causing youths to become dysfunctional in everyday thought processing. When thought processes are altered, many youths operate in an unstated context of conventional thought that obscures or avoids acknowledging how the world is. This is especially true of youth choices, once marijuana abuse sets in. Self-deception is the basis of in-authenticity among youths who abuse marijuana: living that is not based on the truth of oneself in the world leads to dread, guilt, and anxiety. Gestalt therapy provides a way of being authentic and meaningfully responsible for oneself. By becoming aware, one becomes able to choose and/or organize one's own existence in a meaningful manner (Jacobs, 1978; Yontef, 1982, 1983). Gestalt therapy uses focused awareness and experimentation to achieve insight that may have been lost as a result of altered states of mind from youth marijuana abuse. Chapter five examined the Gibson House Experience, emphasizing the hash confrontation in group therapy. The Gestalt method works by engaging in dialogue rather than manipulating the client toward some therapeutic goal. Straightforward caring, warmth, acceptance, and self-responsibility are the hallmark of Gestalt therapy approach. Dialogue in Gestalt group is based on experiencing the other group member as she/he really is and showing the true self, sharing phenomenological awareness. The Gestalt group leader says what she/he means and means what she/he says and encourages group members to do the same. This type of dialogue embodies authenticity and responsibility. Four characteristics of dialogue are emphasized in the Gestalt therapeutic relationship:

- Inclusion – This is putting oneself as fully as possible into the experience of the other without judging, analyzing, or interpreting while simultaneously retaining a sense of one's separate, autonomous presence. This is an existential and interpersonal application of the phenomenological trust in immediate experience. Inclusion provides an environment of safety for the client's phenomenological work and by communicating an understanding of the client's experience, helps sharpen the client's self-awareness.
- Presence – The Gestalt therapist expresses her/himself to the client. Regularly, judiciously, and with discrimination she/he expresses observations, preferences, feelings, personal experience, and thoughts. Thus, the therapist shares her

perspective by modeling phenomenological reporting, which aids the client's learning about trust and use of immediate experience to raise awareness. If the therapist relies on theory-derived interpretation, rather than personal presence, she leads the client into relying on phenomena not in his own immediate experience as the tool for raising awareness. In Gestalt therapy the therapist does not use presence to manipulate the client to conform to pre-established goals, but rather encourages clients to regulate themselves autonomously.

- Commitment to dialogue – Contact is more than something two people do to each other. Contact is something that happens between people, something that arises from the interaction between them. The Gestalt therapist surrenders her/himself to this interpersonal process. This allows contact to happen rather than manipulating, making contact, and controlling the outcome.

- Dialogue is lived – Dialogue is something done rather than talked about. "Lived," emphasizes the excitement and immediacy of doing. The mode of dialogue can be dancing, singing, talking or any modality that expresses and moves the energy between or among the participants. An important contribution of Gestalt therapy to phenomenological experimentation is enlarging the parameters to include explication of experience by nonverbal expressions. However, the interaction is limited by ethics, appropriateness, therapeutic tasks, and so on.

It is important for youth addiction counselors to understand that dialogue does not necessarily mean reliving the counselor's own drug use experience. One common problem among inexperienced youth counselors as we saw in chapter four is the tendency for youth counselors to self disclose their personal addiction experience in the hope that youths will understand the counselors themselves "have been there, done that." Many youths do not receive self-disclosures from counselors well. Often, the beginning counselor who attempts to use the Gestalt approach during group counseling imagines that by self-disclosing her/his drug use experience, she/he may be adding dimension to the phenomenological explication of the group dialogical experience. While few youths may appreciate such kind gestures, others perceive it as loopholes in their natural status quo. Some youths, especially those still wallowing in denial, see self-disclosure as an avenue for future challenge to the counselor's credibility. One Job Corps youth counselor intern once did a very touchy self-disclosure in an attempt to add dimension and phenomenological experimentation to group discussion. After her wonderful revelation, she asked for feedback from the group. One of the female youth bluntly told her that her testimony was 'nice and all,' but added she (the counselor intern) was stupid to have stayed in addiction that long. Another youth added: "it seems like you had your fun, back in the days, before things turned on you. So, why are you always sweating us when we ask for weekend pass?" Group discussion for that particular session took a nosedive to the wrong direction. The general rule of thumb in Gestalt therapy when working with youths is to process experience and not explanation. When experience is processed, insight is gained. Applebaum, a psychoanalyst, observed:

> In Gestalt Therapy the patient quickly learns to make
> the discrimination between ideas and ideation, between
> well-worn obsessional pathways and new thoughts,
> between a statement of experience and not explanation,
> based on the belief that insight which emerges as the
> Gestalt emerges is more potent than insight given by
> the therapist, does help the patient and therapist draw
> and maintain these important distinctions. (1976, p.
> 757)

Gestalt therapy can be used effectively with any client population that the therapist understands and feels comfortable with. If the therapist can relate to the client, the Gestalt therapy principles of dialogue and direct experiencing can be applied. With each client, general principles must be adopted to the particular clinical situation. If the client's treatment is made to conform to Gestalt therapy, it can be ineffective or harmful. A schizophrenic, a sociopath, a borderline, and an obsessive-compulsive neurotic may all need different approaches. Thus, the competent practice of Gestalt therapy requires a background in more than Gestalt therapy. Knowledge of diagnosis, personality theory, and psychodynamic theory is also needed. The individual clinician has a great deal of discretion in Gestalt therapy. Modifications are made by the individual therapist, according to therapeutic style, personality, diagnostic considerations, and so on. This encourages and requires individual responsibility by the therapist. Gestalt therapists are encouraged to have a firm grounding in personality theory, psychopathology, and theories and applications of psychotherapy, as well as adequate clinical experience. Participants in the therapeutic encounter are encouraged to experiment with new behavior and then share cognitively and emotionally what the experience was like. First, clients may be required to go back to old behaviors *then* before exploring new behavior, *now*. Shuttling clients between now and then can present a unique challenge. Because of the impact of Gestalt therapy and the ease with which strong, frequently buried affective reactions can be reached, it is necessary to establish "safe islands" to which both the therapist and client can comfortably return. It is imperative for the therapist to stay with the client until she/he is ready to return to these safety islands. For example, after an especially emotional laden experience, the client may be encouraged to make visual, tactile, or other contact with the therapist or with one or more group members and report the experience. Another safety technique is to have the client shuttle back and forth between making contact in the now with the therapist or group members and with the emotionally laden unfinished situation that the patient was experiencing then until all of the affect has been discharged and the unfinished situation worked through.

Gestalt therapy is very effective with marijuana-impaired youths. These youths generally like to manipulate others. Many adults who work with such youths experience frustration. The more frustration the adult feels and exhibits, the more control youths feel, the weaker the therapeutic alliance, and the more youths fulfill their wishes of not responding to treatment. The scenario accounts for the high recidivism in many youth treatment program. Gestalt therapy balances frustration and support. The therapist explores rather than gratifies the youth client's wishes. This is frustrating to the youth. When this happens, the youth becomes aware of her/his own action in relation to others. Providing contact to the youth is supportive, although this honestly frustrates the youth's manipulative moves. The gestalt therapy expresses self and emphasizes exploring, including exploring desire, frustration, and indulgence. The therapist responds to manipulations by the youth without reinforcing them, without judging, and without being purposely frustrating. The youth, in turn, is surprised at the therapist's stoical warmth – a gesture that defies the youth's devilish expectation and eventually forces the youth to re-examine her/his own tolerance of reverse frustration. This act of balancing warmth with firmness makes the youth to take charge of her/his life. The therapist facilitates attention to opening restricted awareness and areas of constricted contact boundaries. As sensing of failed manipulation increases in accuracy and vividness, as denial is faced with objective evaluation and less resistance, and as youths makes better contact with the therapist, they bring the skill of therapy into their lives. The Gestalt therapy emphasis on personal responsibility, interpersonal contact, and increased clarity of awareness of what is, eventually subjects the youth to face and resolve her/his repressed problems in the present. Suddenly, the youth gains insight into her/his problem as other group members begin to give feedbacks and share their own experiences.

Generally, Gestalt therapy groups last from one and one-half to three hours in length with an average length of two hours. Youths tend to have short attention span. It may be best to start off a youth group therapy to last for about fifty minutes to one hour until the group begins to feel strong contact and support. Once youths allow themselves to become enmeshed in the group process, they usually will go one and one-half hour to two, but group cohesion tend to disintegrate after two hours. As was noted earlier in chapter five, youths are generally reluctant to bring their problem to group discussion. One way to reduce the reluctance is to conduct a one-on-one therapy in the group setting. There is always the one youth who is not afraid to talk freely about her/his problem. The therapist should identify that one youth and use the youth to bait others into group process. Typically, the therapist asks the willing youth if she/he will like to discuss a particular problem in group. The youth is put on a 'hot seat' and an extended interaction ensues between the youth and the therapist or counselor. During the one-on-one contact, the other group members remain silent. At the end of the interaction, group members are asked to give feedback on how they were affected, what they observed, and how their own experiences are similar to those their peer worked on. Oftentimes, this approach starts the ball rolling. Other youths begin to schedule themselves for subsequent sessions, which last between 20 to 30 minutes with additional 15 to 20 minutes for feedback. As the one-on-one therapy in group setting gather momentum and most youths in the group gets a chance to deal with their issues, a skilled therapist may revert to group therapy. By this time, group cohesion has already begun. The 'terminally super unique' youths have been suffocated with warmth and support from the therapist, and for the most part those youths have become the outcast in the group – something youths don't usually like to be. At this stage of the group development, a mild coercion is in place and tolerance for chaotic or nuisance behavior is wearing thin. As group therapy formation progresses, late bloomers seek attention by requesting one-on-one resolution to their problem. Those types of requests are, for the most part, a last minute desperate attempt to disrupt the flow of the group, rather than an honest request to deal with issues. Again, a clinically savvy therapist/counselor acknowledges the request with "warmth that kills." The renegade youth is left bare to come forth with her/his real or imagined issue for discussion. Occasionally, the youth apologizes in the middle of discussion for tabling a non-existent problem, to the dismay of her/his peers, and offers to deal with a real issue. Once again, the veteran therapist offers apology to the group on behalf of the terminally unique renegade and patiently starts over. One thing leads to another, but real progress is made as resistance to group process is torn down. Finally, a cohesive group with greater fluidity and flexibility is formed. Emphasis at this stage is greater involvement and interrelationship or contact in the group. The group leader may choose to use structured or no structured group exercises, while observing the group evolve to its own structure. Often the group begins with some exercise to help group members make the transition into working by sharing here-and-now experience.

Although no suggestion is made that Gestalt therapy is the only or best method for youth group process, it certainly stands out from other psychotherapeutic approaches. We must continue to emphasize that eclectic grill calls for the use of varied methods when working with youths or any addicted population. One must not leave this section of the book feeling like the Gestalt therapy has the key that unlocks treatment of marijuana impaired youths. However, when compared with other psychotherapeutic techniques, Yontef (1969) noted that:

> The theoretical distinction between Gestalt Therapy, behavior modification and psychoanalysis is clear. In behavior modification, the patient's behavior is directly changed by the therapist's manipulation of environmental stimuli. In psychoanalytic theory, behavior is caused by unconscious motivation which becomes manifest in the transference relationship. By analyzing the transference the repression is lifted, the unconscious becomes conscious. In Gestalt Therapy the patient learns to fully use his internal and external senses so he can be self-responsible and self-supportive. Gestalt Therapy helps the patient regain the key to this state, the awareness of the process of awareness. Behavior modification conditions (by) using stimulus control, psychoanalysis cures by talking about and discovering the cause of mental illness (the problem), and Gestalt Therapy brings self- realization through Here-and-now experiments in directed awareness. (pp. 33-34)

When youths become addicted to marijuana, they loose touch with reality, as we know it. They form hardcore defense mechanisms that over a long period become their reality. What may have started off as defense mechanism or denial or repressed memory eventually takes on a life of its own. The addicted youth gradually transitions from the pains associated with the underlying causes of her/his addiction reality to an illusion of uniqueness – one that is marked by a distorted sense of the real world and lack of authenticity. Gestalt therapy offers restoration of the real world insight through the therapist, who models this reality base with integrity, warmth, contact and authenticity. In fact, Levitsky and Simkin (1972) illustrates this point:

> If we were to choose one key idea to stand as a symbol
> for the Gestalt approach, it might well be the concept
> of authenticity, the quest for authenticity...if we regard
> therapy and the therapist in the pitiless light of
> authenticity, it becomes apparent that the therapist
> cannot teach what he does not know...a therapist with
> some experience really knows within himself that he is
> communicating to his patient his (the therapist's) own
> fears as well as his courage, his defensiveness as well
> as his clarity. The therapist's awareness, acceptance,
> and sharing of these truths can be a highly persuasive
> demonstration of his own authenticity. Obviously such
> a position is not acquired overnight. It is to be learned
> and relearned ever more deeply and not only
> throughout one's career but throughout one's entire
> life. (pp. 251-252)

ALTERNATE TREATMENT APPROACHES

The illusive nature of addictive disorder makes it difficult, sometimes, to pinpoint exactly what was effective in treating or forcing addiction to remission. In recent times, many alternate treatment approaches claiming to 'cure' addiction have emerged. Some are questionable, some ephemerally prod food for thought, while others conjure controversy. Our primary premise of contention is that through eclectic approach, we are able to attain a more lasting result than we would, should we strictly adopt a specific treatment protocol. Several years ago, while working with the Job Corps youths, some youths complained about not being able to sleep during acute detoxification. The author being an avid practitioner of yoga decided to introduce yoga Asana (physical exercise) to address the problem of sleeplessness. The result was instantaneous. Weeks later a complete physical fitness program was designed as an offshoot of the yoga experience. So, while we question the validity of alternate treatment approaches, we must keep an open mind to their intended purpose. Until we are able to narrow down the exact causes of addiction, and correspondingly isolate a specific treatment for it, we must continue to use varied methods to treat addiction. One alternate treatment approach that heralded international controversy was the Swiss Heroin Project epitomized as the apogee of Harm Reduction alternate treatment approach. Harm Reduction is not a new concept in treatment, but when it came to prescribing pure pharmaceutical grade heroin to a large number of addicts under a clinical setting sponsored by the Swiss government, global moral majority voiced their opinions. The result of the Swiss Heroin Project received a bi-polar opinion on what constituted treatment success. The following except on Harm Reduction is taken from *Anthology of Monographs on Addiction Studies*:

HARM REDUCTION – A RATIONAL COMPROMISE

The failure of prohibition and traditional substance abuse treatment services to obliterate the pernicious cankerous effect of drug abuse prompted proponents of harm reduction to believe that it is better to take measures to reduce the harm associated with drug use. The harm reduction approach, which is based on public health principles, avoids the extremes of value-loaded judgments on drug use and focuses on the reduction of drug-related harm through pragmatic and low-threshold programs. According to Sally Satel, "Its advocates present harm reduction as a rational compromise between the alleged futility of the drug war and the extremism of outright legalization. But since harm reduction makes no demand on addicts, it consigns them to their addiction, aiming only to allow them to destroy themselves in relative 'safety' – and at taxpayers expense. "[1] At the conceptual level harm reduction maintains a value-neutral humanistic view of drug use and the user, focuses on problems rather then on use per se, neither insists on nor objects to abstinence and acknowledges the active role of the user in harm reduction programs. At the practical level the aim of harm reduction is to reduce the more immediate harmful consequences of drug use through pragmatic, realistic and low-threshold programs. At the policy level harm reduction generates a hue of acceptable policy measures that match a wide range of drug treatment services and patterns of drug use and problems. Harm reduction models subscribe to abstinence as the ultimate goal of harm reduction. They maintain that there will always be illicit drug use and that many people are simply unwilling or unable to give up drugs entirely but nonetheless could benefit from intervention. Harm reduction proponents argue that small reductions of harm are better than no reduction and definitely better than exacerbation. Robert Westermeyer asserts that harm reduction approaches to addictive behavior are based on three central beliefs:[2]

1. ***Excessive behaviors occur along a continuum of risk ranging from minimal to extreme***. *Addictive behaviors are not all-or-nothing phenomena. Though a drug or alcohol abstainer is at risk of less harm than a drug or alcohol user, a moderate drinker is causing less harm than a binge drinker; a crystal methamphetamine smoker or sniffer is causing less harm than a crystal injector.*
2. ***Changing addictive behavior is a stepwise process, complete abstinence being the final step***. *Those who embrace the harm reduction model believe that any movement in the direction of reduced harm, no matter how small, is positive in and of itself.*
3. ***Sobriety isn't for everybody***. *Bold and radical, this statement requires the acceptance that many people live in horrible circumstances. Some are able to cope without the use of*

---

[1] *Satel, Sally. "Opiates For The Masses," Wall Street Journal. June 8, 1998*
[2] *Westermeyer, Robert W. "Reducing Harm Reduction: A Very Good Idea."*
September 18, 2000. http://www.cts.com/crash/habtsmrt/harm.html p. 1-2

drugs, and others use drugs as a primary means of coping. Until we are in a position to offer an alternative means of survival to these folks, we are in no position to cast moral judgment. Westermeyer added that "it is held that the health and well-being of the individual is of primary concern; if individuals are unwilling or unable to change addictive behavior at this time, they should not be denied services. Attempts should be made to reduce the harm of their habits as much as possible." Harm Reduction may sound novel, but its application dates back 30 years. The New York City Health Research Counsel in an attempt to counter discouraging treatment outcome for heroin users began to investigate Methadone as a viable treatment option for heroin dependents. The Nixon administration boosted the number of methadone clinic across the U.S. At the same period, the FDA and DEA set minimum standards for methadone administration.[3] P.G. Erickson observes three phases of the development of harm reduction:[4] The first phase stemmed from a growing concern in the 1960s about the health risks associated with tobacco and alcohol use in the population. The second phase began in 1990 with a sharp focus on AIDS prevention among injection drug users. He states that we have now reached the third phase, in which an integrated public health perception is being developed for all licit and illicit drugs. In this new phase more and more new topics pertaining to harm reduction model are being explored. These topics include small harm reduction such as condom distribution, needle exchange, to total harm reduction such as methadone therapy and outright heroin prescription. White, (1998), contend that "harm-reduction strategies in the modern era have included recommendations for public funding of 'wet hotels,' where chronic inebriates could be supervised

---

[3] *Westermeyer, Robert W. Methadone Maintenance: "The Grandfather of Harm Reduction."* http://www.cts.com/crash/habtsmrt/methad.html *p. 1*
[4] *Erickson, P.G. "Introduction: The Three Phases of Harm Reduction Movement. An examination of Emerging Concepts, Methodologies, and Critiques. Substance Use Misuse. 1999, vol.34, p. 1-7*

minimally, in order to reduce their disruptiveness and cost to the community, and the provision of drug information that would help drug users achieve lower-risk methods of use." He added "By far the most controversial of recent proposals were the provision of information on safer methods of drug injection and the provision of sterile needles to addicts."[5] Proponents of harm reduction maintain that harm reduction eliminates the sequelae of drug abuse to society and to the addict. Opponents sometimes accuse proponents of harm reduction of enabling drug addicts and setting the stage for drug legalization. The debate over harm reduction, legalization and prohibition should continue, so that existing drug strategies will be constantly re-evaluated and reviewed for improvement. (pp. 12-17)

The CAB Health & Recovery Services in collaboration with the Essex County Juvenile Court in Massachusetts uses harm reduction model in their youth-specific (7 to 17) treatment program. Messages such as no drinking and driving, no pot use during school hours, or no hard drugs use are conveyed to youths as part of the program treatment philosophy. The program clinical treatment services director, Michael Levy, Ph.D. writes: "Talk with adolescents about their peer group. They may report that 'all my friends are doing drugs,' but further discussion may reveal that some friends are more heavily involved than others. If a complete change of peer group is impossible, your client may be encouraged to try to stay away from these heavy users in favor of friends who use more occasionally." Ironically, those heavy users may have been occasional users at some point in time. Such is the nature of addiction.

A more recent alternate treatment approach is the use of medication to treat addiction. Counseling alone sometimes falls short of treating severe damages caused by addiction or fails to stop the addicted from further indulgence. As more research in the area of the brain reveals new information, we are beginning to see the use of pharmacologic drugs such as the Selective Serotonin Re-uptake

---

[5] *White, William L. p. 292*

Inhibitors in treatment of addiction. In fact, there is a growing trend in the use of drugs to treat addiction. The use of drugs to treat addiction was initially limited to detoxification. Since the middle 1990s, it has become more common to treat addictive disorders with medicinal drugs – a trend that addiction counselors of the past generation would have found repulsive. This century promises a broad range of drugs in the treatment of addiction. The development of highly selective, receptor site-specific designer drugs and innovative therapies may enhance opiate function and revolutionize mental health. According to an article written by Kim Roller: "What we are seeing is that medication treatment is more and more into mainstream for substance abuse," said Dr. Betty Tai of the National Institute of Drug Abuse, a division of the National Institute of Health. Dr. Tai added that in the past, practitioners have used medication to relieve symptoms – intoxication, overdosing, or withdrawal, using off-label anecdotally. Right now, he said, it is time to systematically develop medication that are specifically for the purpose of treatment.

Systematic de-sensitization is yet another alternate treatment. This model promises to help clients sustain a successful recovery process by extinguishing their craving for alcohol and drugs. The model is currently marketed as Exposure Response Prevention (ERP). ERP claims to be a cue-exposure, cognitive behavioral therapy procedure that systematically exposes an addict to simulated versions of their drugs of choice and the equipment they use to prepare and consume them; is based on sound and well-researched behavioral intervention methodologies; helps to inoculate clients against craving and assists them in managing their relapse triggers; and is an eclectic treatment that is compatible with 12 step programs. The fundamental philosophy of systematic de-sensitization technique is that by constantly and progressively (from mild to severe stimuli) exposing addicts to their drug use triggers, they become de-sensitized to those triggers and thereby are able to block euphoric recalls, which lead to relapses. We will examine in nutshell five other alternate treatment approaches. Again, none of these treatment approaches is endorsed as cure for addiction, but instead to expose a variety of treatment tools in contemporary treatment armamentarium. What follows below is a short synopsis of various alternate treatments for addiction taken from

Counselor (June 2003) magazine, written by William A. Howatt, Ph.D. and Robert H. Coombs, Ph.D.

- **Autogenetic training (AT)** teaches clients how to lower their daily stress level. It is a systematic program that helps both mind and body relax, thereby, enabling the person to return to a normal state. To the external observer, AT may resemble meditation, progressive muscle relaxation, or visualization. However, the internal process utilizes body sensations (e.g., person focuses on a left arm feeling heavy) as the antecedent to the healing state (mild trance). AT teaches a person what is referred to as "self-regulation." The person is taught how to use their mind to directly influence their body's self-regulative systems: circulation, breathing, heart rate, etc. This strategy can reduce the damage of the fight or flight response. According to the writers research suggests AT can be effective as hypnosis in reducing stress and anxiety.
- **Neurolinguistic Programming (NLP)** involves changing a person's perception. This process can be used to assist people with craving that involve the five senses (sight, smell, taste, touch and hearing). For example, a person who craves chocolate can be taught to change their perception of the chocolate experience. The client is first asked to choose two items: the food they want to stop craving, (for example, chocolate), and a food they dislike (for example, eggs). Then the counselor uses a checklist to survey the sub-modalities, stored by the senses, for each food. The client might be asked several questions detailing visual associations for chocolate. There are 30 questions for each food, involving each sense. Once sub-modalities are collected, the client is asked to recall, for example, the visual sub-modalities of chocolate, and replace them with the visual sub-modalities of many eggs. This technique ruins chocolate for some for a long time. This technique claims to have good success with smokers.
- **Self-hypnosis** happens without a hypnotist, but offers the same benefits as traditional hypnosis: stress reduction, relaxation, and stimulation of the body's natural repair system

(Alman and Lamrou, 1992). A counselor oversees the preparation steps, which entails developing a script – a story containing the suggestions the client wishes to ingrain in their sense of being. Once this is accomplished, the client may then begin work on her/his own self-hypnosis tape. Before starting, the individual is taught guided imagery and encouraged to find a place where they feel safe practicing it. Progressive muscle relaxation also is taught to help the person calm down sufficiently to start the process. Ultimately the person goes to their chosen quiet spot, settles down with some progressive muscle relaxation, and turns on the tape to begin their self-hypnosis.

- **Thought Field Therapy (TFT)** is a process that stimulates acupuncture meridians through the light tapping of meridian sites (Callahan, 1995). The area tapped is dictated by the client's concern. The cure for craving, for example, suggests 20 taps under the eye with both hands (Gallo, 1999). The originator, Dr. John Callahan, also developed a set of protocol for dealing with what he defines as psychological reversals, i.e., to help clients align their motivation along with conscious desires. The client will normally be instructed to tap with only two fingers – index and middle. In addition, the counselor using TFT will use the technology of applied person, which result in the experience of negative emotions. The most prominent study on the effectiveness of TFT was conducted by Carbonell and Figley (1999), which suggested TFT is an effective intervention for emotional discomfort.

- **Timeline Therapy (TLT)** focuses on influencing the client's temporal experience and changing her/his view of negative life experiences. TLT provides the client a framework with which to address past issues. Detail, facts, and painful emotions are not rehashed, because in this model there is no need to know them. TLT presents the client's entire past as a metaphor that informs their temporal experience. The goal is to release negative emotions that have remained troubling in the present. The client is invited to change their understanding of the past negative emotions and limiting the decisions these events precipitated. TLT can assist people with depression, anxiety, and other emotional concerns such as anger, so that they can move forward and create the future they really want.

RATIONAL-EMOTIVE APPROACH

Albert Ellis developed rational-emotive behavior therapy in the early 1950s. Ellis' method of psychotherapy works well with juvenile delinquents, truants and youths with sexual difficulties and straight psychotic, including those with delusions and hallucinations, when they are somewhat in contact with reality. This psychotherapy technique uses cognitive-behavior therapy method. The crux of this technique lies in the therapist ability to recognize the belief system and thought pattern that cause clients distress or anxiety. The therapist then helps the clients dispute or dispel those belief systems or thought patterns, and possibly learn new, more healthy belief systems or though patterns. The underlying assumption is that our belief system, which powers our attitudes and expectation influence our reaction to internal and external stimuli. In other words, it is not the activating events (A) of a person's live that cause dysfunctional emotional consequences (C); instead, it is that the person interprets those events unrealistically and therefore have irrational beliefs (B) about them. Rational-emotive therapy worked well with marijuana impaired youths who were also gang members. Many of these youths have similar stories. Typically, the story goes something like this: "My dad left me when I was three years old, or my mom was hooked on drugs and could not provide for me and my sisters, or my uncle sexually abused me when I was 13 years old, etc." In time, these youths are recruited by other youths that have undergone the same plight and together they develop irrational defensive set of survival values that are self-defeating at the long run. They form an attitude of "them against us." They see parents and society as the enemy and see themselves as victims who will not amount to much because of the wrong done to them by the "enemies.' Accordingly, Ellis believes that people are born with predisposition to be either rational or irrational, and that mental disturbances are the product of faulty learning. Here we see that it is not only the events in the youth's life, but also the youth's interpretation of those events that can cause psychological disturbances. Interestingly enough, there is another underlying assumption here, which is, that since mental disorders are the result of learning, they can also be unlearned. This second assumption is what Rational-emotive therapy tries to accomplish.

Rational-emotive therapy proposes many concepts: *People are born with potential to be rational as well as irrational. * Culture and family group exacerbate people's tendency to irrational thinking, self-damaging, habituations, wishful thinking, and intolerance. Culture and family impact is greatest during early years and consequently people are most influenced by family and social pressure during early life. *Humans tend to perceive, think, emote, and behave simultaneously. They therefore, at one and the same time, are cognitive, affective, and action oriented. They rarely act without also cognizing, because their present sensations or actions are apprehended in a network of prior experiences, memories, and conclusions. They seldom emote without thinking, because their feelings include, and are usually triggered by, an appraisal of a given situation and its importance. They rarely act without perceiving, thinking, and emoting, because these processes provide them with reasons for acting. Therefore, to understand self-defeating conduct, we had better understand how people perceive, think, emote, and act. *Although all the major psychotherapies employ a variety of cognitive, emotive, and desensitizing techniques, and although all may help individuals who have faith and who work at applying them, they are probably not equally effective in terms of time and effort, or in terms of the length of the solution. *Rational-emotive therapists do not believe a warm relationship between counselors and clients is a necessary or significant condition for effective personality change. They believe it is desirable for therapists to fully accept clients but criticize and point out the deficiencies of their behavior. Rational-emotive therapists accept clients as fallible humans without necessarily giving personal warmth. They may use a variety of impersonal therapeutic methods, including didactic discussion, behavior modification, bibliotherapy, audiovisual aids, and activity-oriented homework assignments. *Rational-emotive therapists use role-playing, assertion training, desensitization, humor, operant conditioning, suggestion, and support to help clients.

As A.A. Lazarus (1981) points out in presenting Multi-model therapy, such wide-ranging methods are most effective in helping the client achieve deep-seated cognitive change. Rational-emotive therapy is primarily designed to induce people to examine and change some of their most basic values, especially those values that keep them disturbance prone; and to modify their underlying symptoms-creating propensities. General rational-emotive therapy tends to teach clients rational or appropriate behavior. Preferential rational-emotive therapy teaches clients how to dispute irrational ideas and inappropriate behaviors and to internalize rules of logic and scientific methods. *Rational-emotive therapy holds that virtually all serious emotional problems directly stem from magical, empirically unvalidatable thinking and that if disturbances-creating ideas are vigorously disputed by logical and empirical thinking, they can be eliminated or minimized and will ultimately cease to reoccur. Under this premise it assumed that no matter how defective people's heredity may be, and no matter what trauma they may have experienced, the main reason they now over-react or under-react to obnoxious stimuli (at point A) is that they now have some dogmatic, irrational, unexamined beliefs (at point B). *Rational-emotive technique asserts that insight often do not lead to major personality change because, at best, they help people see that they do have emotional problems and that these problems have dynamic antecedents, presumably in the experiences that occurred during childhood. Accordingly, this kind of insight is largely misleading. It is not the activating events (A) of people's lives that Cause dysfunctional emotional consequences (C); it is that they interpret these events unrealistically and therefore have irrational beliefs (B) about them. The assertion then is that the real cause of upsets, there, is people and not what happens to them (even though the experiences obviously have some influence over what they think and feel). In rational-emotive thinking, insight number 1, namely, that the person's self-defeating behavior is related to antecedent and understandable causes, is duly stressed, but clients are led to see these antecedents largely in terms of past or present activating events.

In individual therapy, the youths generally start off their session by telling their most upsetting feelings or consequences (C) during the first week. The counselor or therapist using rational-emotive therapy technique discovers what activating events (A) occurred before the youth felt so badly and help them see what rational beliefs (rB) and what irrational belief (iB) they held in connection with the activating events. The counselor/therapist teaches the youth to dispute (B) her/his irrational beliefs and give her/him concrete homework activity assignments to help with disputing. The homework is then checked up in the following session, sometime with the help of an RET Self-Help Report Form (Sichel & Ellis, 1984), to see how the youth have tried to use the rational-emotive approach during the week. The counselor/therapist keeps teaching the youth how to dispute her/his irrational beliefs and giving her/him homework assignments until the youth not only start to lose her/his presenting symptoms but acquires a saner, more tolerant attitude towards life. In particular, the counselor/therapist tries to show the youth how: 1. To rid her/himself of anxiety, guilt, and depression by fully accepting her/himself as human beings, whether or not she/he succeeds at important tasks and performances and whether or not people in her/his life approve or love her/him; 2. To minimize her/his anger, hostility, and violence by becoming tolerant of other people even when she/he finds these people's traits or performances unappetizing and unfair, and 3. To reduce her/his low frustration tolerance and inertia by working to change unpleasant reality but learning gracefully to stand it when it is truly inevitable.

Rational-emotive therapy is effective when working with difficult clients. It uses tough love stance and gets confrontational. What would work effectively, Ellis found in the early days of his practice of rational-emotive was an active-directive, cognitive-emotive-behavioristic attack on major self-defeating behavior. The essence of effective psychotherapy according to Ellis is full tolerance of people as individuals combined with a campaign against their self-defeating ideas, traits, and performances. Timothy Moore, writing for the Gale Encyclopedia of Psychology contends that as therapy, rational-emotive therapy is active and sometimes confrontational. Cognitive, emotive, and behavioral methods are used in combination to facilitate client change. Some of the cognitive methods include: disputing irrational beliefs (e.g., pointing out how irrational it would be for a client to believe he/she had to be good at everything in order to consider her/himself worthwhile); thought stopping (the therapist interrupts the maladaptive thought by yelling "STOP"); reframing (situations are looked at from a more positive angle); and problem solving. The emotive techniques, including role-playing, modeling, the use of humor, and shame-attacking exercise, are all aimed at diffusing the upsetting emotions connected with certain behavior or situations. Finally, behavioral techniques such as the use of homework assignments, risk-taking exercises, systematic desensitization (which involves incremental exposure to the frightening situation while focusing on remaining relaxed), and bibliotherapy (reading about the disorder) are all used to teach clients that they can safely and comfortably substitute adaptive behaviors for the maladaptive ones they have relied on in the past.

The main stay of rational-emotive therapy is that emotional upsets, as distinguished from feelings of sorrow, regret, annoyance, and frustrations, are caused by irrational beliefs. These beliefs are irrational because they magically insist that something in the universe should, ought, or must be different from the way it indubitably is. Although these irrational beliefs are ostensibly connected with reality (the activating events at point (A), they are magical ideas beyond the realm of empiricism and are established by arbitrary fiat. They generally take the form of the statement, "Because I want something, it is not only desirable or preferable that it exist, but it absolutely should, and it is awful when it doesn't." No such propositions, obviously, can ever be validated, and yet, oddly enough, such propositions are devoutly held, every day, by literally billions of human beings. That is how incredibly disturbance-prone youths are. Once people become emotionally upset – or, rather, upset themselves – another peculiar thing frequently occurs. Most of the time, they know they are anxious, depressed, or otherwise agitated, and also generally know that their symptoms are undesirable and (in our culture) socially disapproved. They therefore make their emotional consequence (C) or symptom into another activating event (A2) and create a secondary symptom (C2) about this new (A). Thus, if one originally starts with something like (A): "I did poorly on my job today." (B): "Isn't that horrible!" one will wind up with (C): feelings of anxiety, worthlessness, and depression. One may now start all over with (A2): "I feel anxious and depressed, and worthless" (B): "Isn't that horrible!" Now one ends up with C2): even greater feelings of anxiety, worthlessness, and depression. In other words, once one becomes anxious, one frequently makes oneself anxious about being anxious: once one becomes depressed, one makes oneself depressed about being depressed, and so on. One now has two consequences or symptoms for the price of one, and one often goes around and around, in a vicious cycle of condemning oneself for doing poorly at some task, feeling guilty or depressed because of this self-condemnation, condemning oneself for one's feeling of guilt and depression, condemning oneself for condemning oneself, condemning oneself for seeing that one condemns oneself and for still not stopping condemning oneself, condemning oneself for going for psychotherapeutic help and still not getting better, condemning that one is indubitably hopelessly disturbed and that nothing can be done about it: and so on, in an endless spiral.

No matter what the original damning is about – and it hardly matters what it is about, because the activating event (A) is not really that important – one eventually tends to end up with a chain of disturbed reactions only obliquely related to the original traumatic events of one's life. Most psychotherapies concentrate either on (A), the activating events in the individual's life, or on (C), the emotional consequences experienced subsequent to the occurrence of these events, and rarely consider (B), the belief system, which is the vital factor in the creation of disturbance. This is what sets rational-emotive therapy aside from the others – it attempts to dispute the belief system (B). Even, assuming that activating events and emotional consequences are important, there is not too much a counselor/therapist can do by concentrating their therapeutic attention on these two things according to rational-emotive thinking. The activating events are said to belong to the past by the time the counselor/therapist sees the client. Sometimes it was many years ago that the client was abandoned by her/his parents, was sexually abused by her/his uncle, or was neglected by her/his mom. There is nothing anyone can do to change those prior happening from rational-emotive perspective. Ellis believes that as for clients' present feelings, the more we focus on them, the worse they are likely to feel. If we keep talking about the clients' anxiety, getting them to re-experience the feelings, they can easily become more anxious. The most logical point in trying to interrupt their disturbed process is to get them to focus on their anxiety-creating belief system – point (B). If for example, a male client feels anxious during a therapy session and the therapist reassures him that there is nothing for him to be anxious about, he may become more anxious or may achieve a palliative solution to his problem by convincing himself, "I am afraid that I will act foolishly right here and now, and wouldn't that be awful! No, it really wouldn't be awful, because this therapist will accept me anyway.' On the other hand, the therapist can concentrate on the activating events in the client's life, which are presumably making him anxious – by, for instance, showing him that his mother used to point out his deficiencies in making an impression on others, that he was always afraid his teachers would criticize him for reciting poorly, that he is still afraid or speaking to authority figures who might disapprove of him, and that, therefore, because of all his prior and present fears, in situation A1,A2,A3, etc he is now anxious with the therapist. Whereupon the client might convince himself, "Ah! Now I see that I am generally anxious when I am faced with authority figures. No wonder I am anxious even with my own therapist!" In which case, he might feel much better and temporarily lose his anxiety.

It would be much better for the therapist to show this client that he was anxious as a child and is still anxious with various kinds of authority figures not because they are authorities or do have some power over him, but because he has always believed, and still believes, that it is awful when an authority figure disapproves of him, and that he will be destroyed if he is criticized. Whereupon the anxious client would tend to do two things: 1. He would become diverted from (A), criticism by an authority figure, and from (C), his feelings of anxiety, to a consideration of (B), his irrational belief system. This diversion would help him become immediately non-anxious – for when he is focusing on "What am I telling myself (at B) to make myself anxious" he cannot too easily focus upon the self-defeating, useless thought, "Wouldn't it be terrible if I said something stupid to my therapist and if even he disapproved of me!" 2. He would begin actively to dispute (at point D) his anxiety-creating irrational beliefs, and not only could he then temporarily change them (by convincing himself, "It would be unfortunate if I said something stupid to my therapist and he disapproves of me, but it would hardly be terrible or catastrophic!"), but he would also tend to have a much weaker allegiance to these self-defeating beliefs the next time he was with an authority figure and risked criticism by this individual. So he would obtain, by the therapist's getting him to focus primarily on (B) rather than on (A) and (C), curative and prevention, rather than palliative, results in connection with his anxiety. This fore going example is the basic personality theory of rational-emotive therapy: Human beings, for the most part, create their own emotional consequences. They are born with a distinct proneness to do so and learn, through social conditioning, to exacerbate (rather than minimize) that proneness. They nonetheless have considerable ability to understand what they foolishly believe to cause their distress (because they have a unique talent for thinking about their thinking) and to train themselves to change their self-sabotage beliefs (because they also have a unique capacity for self-discipline or self-reconditioning). If they think and work hard at understanding and contradicting their belief system, they can make amazing palliative, curative, and preventive changes in their disturbance-creating tendencies (Ellis, 1978, 1985a, 1987a; Ellis & Dryden, 1987).

We must, again, reemphasize that no one system of psychotherapy is a panacea for 'curing' maladaptive behavior that surface as a result of long time abuse of marijuana by youths. Each psychotherapeutic technique offers a unique solution, but when taken in combination with other methods and alternate treatment systems, a more realistic approach is attained. Rational-emotive behavior therapy when applied to youth treatment, allows a youth to observe, understand, and persistently attack their irrational, grandiose, perfectionist should, ought, and must. It employs the logical and empirical methods of science to encourage youths to surrender resistance, insubordination, pent up anger from the past, and inertia; to acknowledge that nothing is sacred or all-important (although many things are quite important) and nothing is awful or terrible (although many things are exceptionally unpleasant and inconvenient); and to gradually teach themselves and to practice the philosophy of desiring rather than demanding and of working at changing what they can change and gracefully putting up with what they cannot. For what it is worth, rational-emotive therapy efficiently helps youths resist their tendencies to be too unique, disapproving of authority, deviant, and angry at the world at large. It actively and didactically, shows youths how to abet and enhance one side of their social world, while simultaneously changing and living more happily with (and not repressing or squelching) the other side.

SOLUTION FOCUSED THERAPY

In summary, the psychotherapeutic methods and alternate treatment methods chosen here to exemplify what possible mixes there are in the eclectic grill have been randomly selected. There are other methods that are equally or more effective than what has been presented. A youth counselor should choose a method of treatment, based on thorough assessment of a youth's presenting and auxiliary problems. Moreover, it is imperative that whenever possible, a mixture of methods, including the use of medication to reduce the horrific effects of detoxification or to reduce the excruciating phenomenon of craving, be deployed in other to attain the best possible result. Eclecticism challenges treatment professionals, social workers, parents, guardians, teachers, and mentors to abandon some or all of their old ideas when it comes to working with youths (or any population per se) who abuse marijuana or any other drugs. The biggest disservice one can do to a client is to not venture into using proven alternate methods of treatment due to one's bias or professional skepticism, especially when all possible measures have failed in helping the client. The ability to keep an open mind and to, at the very least, investigate other methods of treatment outside of one's treatment comfort zone is the essence of professionalism in our ever-changing world of professional growth. Indeed, as Herbert Spencer once wrote: "There is a principle which is bar against all information, which is proof against all arguments and which cannot fail to keep a man in everlasting ignorance – that principle is contempt prior to investigation," (Alcoholics Anonymous, 2001). We will now examine one more contemporary method of treatment, one that some claim is equally or more effective in working with addicted population – Solution Focused Therapy.

In chapter five we explored the futuristic approach in individual counseling. We noted that once clients can envision a future without drugs, a future full of hope and aspiration and a future that offers something the present does not have, then clients are ready to give treatment a try or at least pay lip service to treatment. Solution Focused Therapy reinforces the same concept. Its fundamental premise is that by focusing on how life will be once the problem is resolved, clients often experience renewed hope that change is possible and that life without the problematic behaviors is desirable. It contends that problems are best understood in relation to their solution (de Shazer, 1985). Contrary to popular beliefs, Solution Focused Therapy is not only for use with clients who have managed care insurance, nor is it a quick fix for mental health problems. It is a model, which evolved over years of thought, research and experience. The Harvard Mental Health Letter (April 1997, vol. 13 Issue 10) suggests Solution Focused Therapy was originally developed by the Family Therapy Center in Milwaukee, and that it uses methods largely adapted from the work of Milton Erickson. Others contend Steve de Shazer and Insoo Kim Berg at the brief Therapy Center in Milwaukee pioneered the approach. Emphasis is placed on respect for clients and their competence, strength and resources in solving their own problems. The important issues are how the client wants things to be different and what it will take to make it happen. It is a system-based model of therapy, which strongly recognizes building a collaborative relationship with the client. In most psychotherapy, clients describe their problems, while therapists ask questions for clarity. The therapists listen attentively with empathy and then discuss the issues at stake with a view to developing alternatives. However, using Solution Focused Therapy, the therapist is required to set her/his own agenda aside and truly listen to what the client wants. This model relies in the expertise of the client to determine what is important to her/him and in turn, allows the client to determine what the client would like to accomplish. This results in partnership with the client and often results in change that is more rapid since the client sees relevance of the treatment to her/his goals. The process is neither exclusively supportive nor exclusively exploratory and insight-oriented. It simply tries to help clients notice how thing would look like when symptoms are diminished or absent and use this knowledge as a foundation for recovery. If a client insists that the symptoms are constant and unrelieved, the therapist works with her/him to find exceptions and make the exceptions more frequent, predictable, and controllable. In other words, therapy builds on working solutions already available to the patient. As a corollary, the therapeutic dialogue is often deliberately diverted from a discussion of the presenting problem(s). This technique challenges the assumption that learning all about the etiology of the problem is the only way to find the solution to the problem, but it is not in competition with traditional or motivational approaches (Taleff, 1997). Motivational approaches are also regarded as a problem solving approach in which the therapist is the 'expert' in identifying a client's issue and resultant treatment plans. By contrast, Solution Focused Therapy advances the notion that there is no single correct or valid way to live one's life, therefore, it is the client's goals, not the therapist's that should be identified and accomplished. Similarly, Solution Focused Therapy supports the four tenants that research indicates cause change (de Shazer, 1985): extra-therapeutic factors (the client's view of the world; therapeutic relationship (the client's perception of the relationship); therapeutic techniques; and expectancy, hope, and placebo factors (Miller, Duncan, & Hubble, 1997).

Solution Focused Therapy uses a thought-provoking question – miracle question – to goad client to explore useful ideas that open up a world of new reality. It also uses other techniques such as pretreatment improvement, noticing difference, exceptions, compliments and scaling to guide clients to problem resolution (Berg & Miller, 1992). We shall examine two of these techniques in the succeeding paragraphs. Typically, the miracle question asks clients to describe, as fully as possible, what they believe their lives would be like without the problem for which they have sought therapy. This question helps the client envision life without the problem. It usually turns out that many clients are so preoccupied with their troubles that they have not given much thought to this question. As a result, "Answering these miracle questions will provide him (the client) with clues on what first steps he needs to take to find solutions and will show him how his life will change, thus giving him hope that his life can change" (Berg, 1994). In asking the miracle question, the therapist serves to help clients identify the inevitable exceptions to the times that they feel troubled. Those exceptions, along with the strengths and resources, which they possess, are used to help clients to help themselves. Solution Focused Therapy is particularly beneficial when working with youths, since it emphasizes the client's strengths and resources, helping the individual apply the skills and strategies that she/he has used successfully in the past. A solution-focused therapist works under the assumption that the client has the answer to her/his problem and the skills and resources needed to resolve it. Focus is placed on the client's view of her/his own concerns (not the therapist's) and on the client's vision for change. Thus, the therapy begins with finding out what the client wants and how she/he will know whether a successful outcome has been reached. This emphasis on the positive and on the client's interpretation of the need for change makes this approach particularly exciting and innovative for dealing with addicted youths. Youths generally want to be in charge and be in control of their destiny. The Solution Focused approach allows youths to be themselves and offer them the opportunity to use the unique street survival skills they had already acquired to solve their own problem. It is a win-win approach for both the therapist and the youth. Instead of the therapist coming across as the agent or initiator of change, she/he comes across as mediator or partner in the change process. The youth is presumably in the driver's seat and not the therapist. The miracle question can be effective with a gangbanging, marijuana impaired youth whose only stated goal is to get off probation. For such a client, the question might be asked like this: "Suppose that a miracle happened while you are asleep tonight. And the miracle is that you have gained the ability to get out and stay out of the legal system. But, since you were asleep, you don't know that the miracle has happened. What will you notice when you wake up that lets you know this miracle has happened?" This question gives the youth the opportunity to explore her/his imagination to great depths. It forces the youth client to honestly examine what life would be like without the presenting problem. Often, this is the key that unlocks the craving for alternative life style. Many youths in course of their addiction and other self-defeating behavior have lost the insight on what everyday life is like. Solution Focused Therapy prods youth to enkindle the zeal to live as most ordinary people do. This, in turn, facilitates the exploration of the youth's current life style and the imminent consequences.

Pretreatment improvement entails asking clients what improvement in their problem have occurred since they got into treatment. The therapist and clients then explore what the clients did to accomplish whatever improvement reported. The unique advantage of this technique is that it helps clients identify what steps they took which produced result, and to further explore such steps by applying them to other arrears of the client's problems. Identifying pretreatment changes may lead clients to feel encouragement because they realize their situation can improve. Research indicates that pretreatment improvement commonly produces result. Allgood, Parham, Salts, & Smith (1995) found that 30% of 200 clients reported pretreatment improvement in the situation that led them to seek therapy. Another study reviewing data from 2400 clients found that 15% made significant improvement before attending their first session (Howard, Kopta, Krause, & Orlinsky, 1986). One interesting report from youths at the Job Corps program regarding pretreatment improvement surrounds the level of control and self-confidence the youths feel from not using drugs during pretreatment activities. The youths usually get a weekend pass to go home two weeks after entering the program. During the two weeks preceding the weekend pass, a lot of time is spent on preparing the youths to go home successfully without a relapse. On return, majority of the youths respond well to pretreatment improvement questions. They overwhelmingly emphasize the excitement of being able to not visit their friends who use drugs, saying no to invitation to use drugs by friends and relatives, and refusing to spend whatever money they go home with on drugs. This element of control over their environment and willpower offers a springboard for further interest in treatment, which leads one to wonder how pretreatment change affect the process and outcome of therapy. One study found that clients who report pretreatment change are four times more likely to complete therapy than clients who clients who report no pretreatment (Johnson, Nelson, Allgood, 1998).

Since the purpose of this book is not to endorse a particular psychotherapeutic method, we will briefly mention the remaining two Solution Focused Therapy questions: With scaling questions, therapists ask a client to rank her/his problem, perception, motivation, prediction, or any clinically relevant issue on a scale of one to ten (de Shazer, 1994). Therapists also ask clients exception questions to identify when the problem was less severe or did not exist and what the client did to accomplish this. Of all four Solution Focused Therapy questions, therapists rated the miracle question as most therapeutic. Scaling questions were the most frequently used and therapists rated these questions as the best way to evaluate a client's progress. Therapists described exception questions as typically leading a client to report exceptions and improvements in her/his problems and to describe what she/he did to achieve the change. Therapists rated questions about pretreatment change as the least effective of the questions and the most difficult to use successfully (Skidmore, 1993). Overall, Solution Focused Therapy is successful with most clients and produces positive outcomes for a variety of clinical problems and in a variety of settings. However, it has been the theme of this book that a cornucopia of therapeutic methods for treating substance abuse and other mental illness abound, and that no one method is a panacea for these problems.

On a final note, because this book focuses on the dangers of marijuana impairment on youths, it is imperative that we revisit the current prevailing trend towards medical marijuana debate. A recent CNN poll suggests that most Americans favor legalizing and taxing marijuana for medical use. The same poll suggests using the tax money from marijuana sales to subsidize rising prescription cost for seniors. Such skewed argument is predicated on erstwhile illogical notion that medical marijuana has been around for nearly 5,000 years and that 34 states, including Washington, D.C. (which combined are home to 70% of the U.S. population) have laws on their books that allow or are otherwise favorable to medical marijuana. Proponents of the medical marijuana chicanery abet their debate by citing illogically that a number of states decriminalized the possession of marijuana long before the most recent California and Arizona initiatives. They purport that Louisiana has passed such a measure three times since 1981, most recently in 1991, and that Virginia has had a similar one on the books since 1979. The recent California law is written so that almost any pain or ailment could be construed as justification for use of marijuana. Proposition 215 also allows the cultivation of marijuana, not just the possession. Arizona's Proposition 200 goes beyond marijuana and empowers doctors to prescribe narcotics such as heroin and LSD, if they see fit. Medical marijuana proponents, who oftentimes use marijuana themselves, summarize their arguments along this lines: Because physicians believe that smoked marijuana is the best available treatment for some of their patients, because smoked marijuana produces no unacceptable risks to its users or the community, because it is half the price of the legal drug marinol (which works similarly to smoked marijuana for some patients) and because 70% of the U.S. population wants it as a medical option, smoked marijuana should be a medical option now. One of the inherent problems with smoked marijuana, as with most psychoactive substances, is that once under the influence of marijuana, it is difficult to discern objective reality from distorted fact. Many proponents of medical marijuana laws lack the objective reality to fully assess the real dangers and implications of legalizing marijuana for medical use. Medical marijuana proponents are challenged to visit the clinical minds of marijuana-impaired youths. Well, what difference will it make if they are in the same frame of mind as the youth themselves? As was stated in chapter three, they (medical marijuana proponents) are probably feeling "terminally unique" in advancing propositions that defy the physician's first rule – *primum non nocere*. The physician's first rule is that whatever treatment a physician prescribes to a patient – first, that treatment must not harm the patient.

What is at stake with medical marijuana is not whether marijuana can alleviate symptoms of particular ailments, but instead, the degree of harm associated with its use. It is medical antithesis to cure glaucoma and harm the lungs, or to alleviate pain at the expense of weakening the immune system. Sure smoked marijuana may contain THC, which may help arrest nausea, but it also has 400 other chemicals and oxidants, which may harm the lungs, brain, T-cells, and motor skills. Marinol is a safe alternative to smoked marijuana. This is a fact that has fallen on the deaf ears of medical marijuana proponents. In fact, the California Narcotics Officers Association, in their policy statement "The Use of Marijuana as a Medicine," published on their website as of May 22, 2002, noted: "Marinol differs from the crude plant marijuana because it consists of one pure, well-studied, FDA-approved pharmaceutical in stable known dosages. Marijuana is an unstable mixture of over 400 chemicals which are largely unstudied and appear in uncontrolled strengths." Even the American Medical Association (AMA) believes that the National Institute of Health (NIH) should use its resources and influence to support the development of a smoke-free inhaled delivery system for marijuana or THC to reduce the health hazards associated with the combustion and inhalation of marijuana. The AMA calls for further adequate and well-controlled studies of marijuana and related cannabinoids in patients who have serious conditions for which preclinical anecdotal, or controlled evidence suggests possible efficacy and the application of such results to the understanding and treatment of disease. The AMA recommends that marijuana be retained in Schedule I of the controlled Substance Act pending the outcome of such studies. The U.S. Drug Enforcement Administration (DEA) published in its website in February 2003 that "Not one American health association accepts marijuana as medicine."

Many prescription drugs are currently abused. If smoked marijuana becomes a legal prescription drug, it will have its fair share of abuse. This time not only by adults who manipulate doctors, but also by youths who are already prone to the drug use culture. Medical marijuana will have far-reaching consequences on the overall health our youths. Marijuana is notorious for its gateway properties. Legalizing marijuana for medical purposes will definitely not eliminate its gateway propensity. In fact, it will enhance the tendency for proponents of drug legalization to want to push for medical LSD, cocaine, methamphetamine, heroin, ad infinitum. Arizona's

Proposition 200 already has provision for medical heroin and LSD. Medical marijuana is nothing but red herring for drug legalization and therefore must not be allowed to become legal.

REFERENCES

Ackerman, R.J. Survivors of child abuse and dysfunctional families. Conference Lecture. University of Utah School of Alcoholism and Chemical Dependencies, June 18, 2002.

Ackerman, R.J., Ph.D. Family issues in residential treatment. Conference Lecture. University of Utah School on Alcoholism and Other Drug Dependencies, June 17, 2002.

Adolescent self-reported behaviors and their association with marijuana use. SAMHSA 1998. Based on the data from the National Household Survey on Drug Abuse, 1994-1996.

Alcoholics Anonymous, (1939). The story of how more than one hundred men have recovered from alcoholism. First Edition. New York: Works publishing Company.

Alcoholics Anonymous, (2001). Fourth Edition. New York: Alcoholics Anonymous World Services, INC.

Allgood, S.M., Parham, K.B., Salts, C.J., & Smith, T.A. (1995). The association between pretreatment change and unplanned termination in family therapy. The American Journal of Family Therapy, 23.

Appelbaum, S.A. (1976). Psychoanalyst looks at gestalt therapy. In C. Hatcher & P. Himelstein (Eds.). The handbook of gestalt therapy. New York: Jason Aronson.

Bandura, A. (1969). Principles of behavior modification. New York: Holt, Rinehart and Winton.

Bandura, A. (1977). A social learning theory. Englewood Cliffs, N.J.: Prentice Hall.

Bandura, A. (1986). Social foundations of thought and action: A social cognitive theory. Englewood Cliffs, N. J: Prentice Hall.

Barnett, M. L (1955). Alcoholism in the Cantonese of New York City: An anthropological study. In O. Diethalin (Eds.). Etiology of Chronic Alcoholism. Springfield, IL: Charles C. Thomas.

Barton, J., Chassin, L., & Presson, C.C. (1982). Social image factors as motivators of smoking initiation in early and middle adolescence. Child Development, 53: 1499-1511.

BBC News, (June 24, 1998). Genetic link to smoking addiction. http://news.bbc.co.uk/hi/english/health/newsid_119000/119442. stm.

Beatty, L. Ph.D. Effective therapies for minorities: Meeting the need of racially and culturally different clients in substance-abuse treatment (pp.37). Counselor, October 2000.

Beatty, L., Ph.D. Effective therapies for minorities: Meeting the needs of racially and culturally different clients in substance abuse treatment. Counselor, October 2000, pp. 37.

Begleiter, H., Porjesz, B., Bihari, B. & Kissin, B. (1984). Event-related brain potentials in boys at risk for alcoholism. Science, vol. 225:1493-1496.

Berg, I.K. & Miller, S.D. (1992). Working with the problem drinker: A solution-focused approach. New York: Norton.

Berg, I.K. (1994). Family based services: A solution-focused approach (pp. 100). New York: Norton.

Bertalanffy, L. Von, (1974). General systems theory and psychiatry. In S. Arieti (Eds.), American Handbook of Psychiatry, (vol. 1, pp. 1095-1117). New York: Basic Books.

Bigelow, G., Liebson, I. & Griffith, R. (1974). Alcoholic drinking: Suppression by a brief time-out procedure. Behavior Restoration Therapy, vol. 12: 107-115.

Bohman, M. (1978). Some genetic aspects of alcoholism and criminality. Archives of General Psychiatry. Vol. 35:269-276.

Borgatta, E.F. & Lambert, W.W. (1968). (Eds.) Counseling and psychotherapy. Handbook of personality theory and research. Chicago, IL: Rand McNally.

Bradshaw, J. (1989). Healing the shame that binds you. Dearfield Beach, Florida: Health Communications, Inc.

Burton, A. (1969). Encounter. San Francisco: Jossey-Bass.

Cadoret, R.J. & Cain, C. (1980). Sex differences in predictors of antisocial behavior in adoptees. Archives of General Psychiatry.

Cadoret, R.J., & Gath, A. Inheritance of alcoholism in adoptees. British Journal of Psychiatry. Vol. 132:252-258.

Cahalan, D. & Room, R. (1974). Problem drinking among American men. Rutger Center of Alcohol Studies Monographs, No. 7, New Brunswick, NJ.

Chaplin, J.P. (1985). Dictionary of psychology. New York: Dell
Publishing.

Christen, J.A., & Christen, A.G., (1992). Combined tobacco and
alcohol addiction: A prototypic form of poly-drug use.
Indianapolis, IN: Indiana University School of Dentistry.

Clark, W.B. & Cahalan, D. (1976). Changes in drinking over a four-
year span. Addictive Behavior, vol. 1:251-259.

Clononger, C.R., et al. (1978). Implications of sex differences in the
prevalence of antisocial personality, alcoholism, criminality for
family transmission. Archives of General Psychiatry, vol. 35:941-
951.

CNN News, (May 20, 1998). Researchers locate areas of a handful of
alcoholism genes.
http://www.cnn.com/HEALTH/9805/20/genetic.alcoholism/.

CNN News, (September 5, 1996). Compulsive gambling a genetic
disorder? http://www.cnn.com/HEALTH/9609/05/born.gambler/.

Cohen, M. Liebson, I.A., Faillace, L.A. & Allen, R.P. (1971).
Moderate drinking by chronic alcoholics: A schedule-dependent
phenomenon. Journal of Nervous Mental Disorder, vol. 153:434-
444.

Corsini, R.J. & Wedding, D. (1989). Current psychotherapies. 4th ed.
Itasca, IL: P.E. Peacock Publishers, Inc.

de Shazer, S. (1988). Investigating solution in brief therapy. New
York: Norton. 1988

de Shazer, S. (1994). Words were originally magic: New York:
Norton.

de Shazer, S. Key to solution in brief therapy. New York: Norton.

Diagnostic and statistical Manual of Mental Disorder. 4th Ed.,
Published by the America Psychiatric Association, Washington,
DC, 1995.

Dole, V.P. Addictive behavior. Scientific American. June 1980.
pp.138-154.

Donegan, N.H. et al. (1983). A learning theory approach to
commonalities. In P.K. Levison, Dr. Gernstein, and Maloff
Lexington (Eds.), commonalities in substance abuse habitual
behavior. MA: Lexington.

Ellis, A. & Dryden, W. (1987). The practice of rational-emotive therapy. New York: Springer.

Ellis, A. (1978). Toward a theory of personality. In R.J. Corsini (Ed.), Readings in current personality theories. Itasca, IL: Peacock.

Ellis, A. (1985a). Overcoming resistance: Rational-emotive therapy with difficult clients. New York: Springer.

Ellis, A. (1987a). A sadly neglected cognitive element in depression. Cognitive Therapy and Research. pp. 11, 121-146.

Erickson, E.H. (1963). Childhood and society. 2nd ed., New York: W.W. Norton and Co., Inc.

Festinger, L. (1957). A theory of cognitive dissonance. Sanford, CA: Stanford University Press.

Fingarette, H., (1970). The perils of powell: In search of a factual foundation for the disease concept of alcoholism. Harvard Law Review, vol. 83: 793-812.

Flores, P.J. (1997). Group psychotherapy with addicted population: An integration of twelve-step and psychodramatic theory. 2nd ed. New York: The Haworth Press. Bernard, H.S. & Mackenzie, K.R. (1994). Basics of group psychotherapy. New York: The Guilford Press.

Fossum, M.A., & Mason, M.J. (1986). Facing shame. New York: W.W. Norton and Co., Inc.

Freud, S. Studies on hysteria. Standard Edition. Vol. 2, 1895.

Freud, S. The neuropsychosis of defense. Standard Edition. Vol. 3, 1894

Gabrielli, W.F., Jr., Mednick, S.A., Volavka, J., Pollock, V.E., Schulsinger, F., & Itil, T.M. (1982). Electroencephalograms in children of alcoholic fathers. Psychology, vol. 19: 404-407.

Gibbons, F.X., Eggleston, T.J., Benthin, A.C. (1997). Cognitive reactions to smoking relapse: The reciprocal relation between dissonance and self-esteem. Journal of Personality and Social Psychology, 72, 184-195.

Goldstein, A. (1976a). Heroin addiction: Sequential treatment employing pharmacological supports. Archives of General Psychology, vol. 33:353-358.

Goldstein, A., (1976b). Opioid (endorphins) in pituitary and brain. Science, vol. 193:1081-1086.

Goodwin, D.W., (1979). Alcoholism and heredity: A review and hypothesis. Archives of General Psychiatry, vol. 36:57-61.

Goodwin, D.W., Crane, J.B., & Guze, S.B. (1971). Felons who drink: An 8-year follow-up. Quarterly Journal of Studies on Alcohol, vol. 32:136-147.

Goodwin, D.W., Schulsinger, F., Hermansen, L., Guze, S.B. & Winokur, G. (1973). Alcohol problem in adoptees raised from alcoholic biological parents. Archives of General Psychology, vol. 28:238-243.

Gusfield, J.R., (1996). Contested meanings: The construction of alcohol problems. Madison, WS: University of Wisconsin Press.

Haggard, H.W., (1944). Critique of the concept of the allergic nature of alcohol addiction. Quarterly Journal of Studies on Alcohol, vol. 5:233-241.

Harding, J.R., (1963). Symbolic crusade: Status politics and the America temperance movement. Champaign, IL: University of Illinoise Press.

Harding, W.M., Zinberg, N.E., Stemack, S.M., & Barry, M., (1980). Formerly-addicted-now-controlled opiate users. International Journal of the Addictions, vol. 15:47-60.

Herdman, J. (1997). Global criteria: The 12 core functions of the substance abuse counselor. 2nd ed.

Horn, D., & Waingrow, S. (1966). Some dimensions of a model for smoking behavior change. American Journal of Public Health, 56:21-26.

Howard, K.I., Lopta, S. M, Krause, M.S., & Orlinsky, D.E. (1986). The dose-effect relationship in psychotherapy. American Psychologist, 41, 159-164.

Howatt, W.A., Ph.D., & Coombs, R.H., Ph.D., New therapeutic approaches: Alternative treatment for addiction. Counselor, June 2003. pp. 4.

Inaba, D.S., & Cohen, W.E. (1989). Uppers, downers, all arounders: Physical and mental effects of psychoactive drugs. Ashland, Oregon: Cinemed, Inc.

Istvan, J., & Matarazzo, J.D., (1984). Tobacco, and caffeine use: A review of their interrelationships. Psychology Bulletin, vol. 95:301-326.

Jackson, J.K., (1958). Types of drinking patterns of male alcoholics. Quarterly Journal of Studies on Alcohol, vol. 19:269-302.

Jacobs, L. (1978). Thou relations in gestalt therapy. In published Doctorial Dissertation. California School of Professional Psychology, Los Angeles.

Jellinek, E.M., (1958). Phases of alcohol addiction. Quarterly Journal of Studies on Alcohol, vol. 13:673-684.

Johnson, L.D., Nelson, T.S. & Allgood, S.M. (1998). Noticing pretreatment change and therapeutic outcomes: An initial study. American Journal of Family Therapy, 26, 159-168.

Knop, et al. (1984). A Danish prospective study of young males at high risk for alcoholism. In D.W. Goodwin, K.T. Van Dusen, and S.A. Mednick (Eds.). Longitudinal research in alcoholism. Boston, MA: Kluwer-Nijhoff.

Kurtz, E., (1979). Not-God: A history of Alcoholics anonymous. Center City, MN: Hazelden Educational Services.

Lazarus, A.A. (1956). A psychological approach to alcoholism. South African Medical Journal, 30, 707-710.

Lazarus, A.A. (1958). New methods in psychotherapy: A case study. South Africa Medical Journal, 32, 660-664.

Lazarus, A.A. (1965). Toward the understanding and effective treatment of alcoholism. South Africa Medical Journal, 39, 736-741.

Lazarus, A.A. (1966). Broad spectrum behavior therapy and the treatment of agoraphobia. Behavior Research and Therapy, 4, 95-97.

Lazarus, A.A. (1971). Behavior therapy and beyond. New York: McGraw-Hill.

Lazarus, A.A. (1981). The practice of multimodel therapy. New York: McGraw-Hill.

Leshner, A.I., Ph.D. Exploring trends in addiction treatment (pp.39). Professional Counselor, October 1998.

Levitsky, A. & Simkin, J.S. (1972). Gestalt therapy. In L.N. Solomon & B. Berzon (Eds.), New perspectives on encounter groups (pp. 245-253). San Francisco: Jossey-Bass.

Levitsky, A., & Simkin, J.S. (1972). Gestalt therapy. In L.N. Solomon & B. Berzon (Eds.). New perspectives on encounter group. San Francisco: Jossey-Bass.

Levy, M., Ph.D. Issues in youth treatment: A more measured, less formal approach. Addiction Professional, March 2003. pp.24.

Lieber, C.S., (1976). Metabolism of alcohol. Scientific America, vol. 234 (No. 3):25-33.

Maddux, J. F & Desmond, D.P., (1981). Career of opioid users. New York: Praeger Publications.

Marlatt, G.A., Demming, B. & Reid, J.B. (1973). Loss of control drinking in alcoholics: An experimental analogue. Journal of Abnormal Psychology, vol. 81:233-241.

Matthew, R., (July 13, 1998). Gene-link breakthrough may explain drug addiction. The Irish Independent. http://www.ukcia.org/news/1998/news/3/st2037.htm.

McCarthy, W., (1985). Date the cognitive developmental model and other alternatives to the social skills deficit model of smoking onset. In C. Bell, & R. Batties (Eds.). Prevention research: Deterring drug abuse among children and adolescents. Washington D.C.: National Institute of Drug Abuse, Government Printing Office.

Mello, N.K. & Mendelson, J.H. (1972). Drinking patterns during work-contingent and non-contingent alcohol acquisition. Psychosomatic Medicine, vol. 34:139-164.

Miller, S. & Rollnick, S. (1991). Motivational interviewing. New York: The Guilford Press.

Miller, S.D., Duncan, B.L., & Hubble, M.A. (1997). Escape from babel: Toward a unifying language for psychotherapy practice (pp. 24-31). New York: Norton.

Miller, W.R. & Rollnick, S. (1991). Motivational interviewing: Preparing people to change addictive behavior. New York: Guilford Press.

Miller, W.R. (2000). Rediscovering Fire: Small interventions, large effects. Psychology of Addictive Behaviors, 14 (1).

Miller, W.R., Brown, J.M., Simpson, T.L., Handmaker, N.S., Bien, T.H., Luckie, L.F., Montgomery, H.A., Hester, R.K. & Tonigan, J.S. (1995). What work? A methodological analysis of the alcohol treatment outcomes literature. In R.K. Hester & W.R. Miller (Eds.), Handbook of alcoholism treatment approaches: Effective alternatives. Boston, MA: Allyn & Bacon.

Miller, W.R., Zweben, A., DiClemente, C.C., & Rycharik, R.G. (1992). Motivational enhancement therapy manuel: A clinical research guide for therapists treating individuals with alcohol abuse and dependence (NIAAA Project MATCH Monograph, vol. 2. DHHS Publication No. ADM 92-1894). Washington D.C.: U.S. Government Printing Office.

Monitoring the Future, 2001.

Moore, T. Rational-emotive behavior therapy. Gale encyclopedia of Psychology. http://www.findarticle.com/cf._0/g2699/005/2699000599/p1/articl e.jhtml/?term = rational +. Retrieved September 30, 2003.

Moreno, J.L. Psychodrama. New York: Beacon, vols. 1-3, 1946-1969.

National Household Survey on Drug Abuse, 2000.

National Household Survey on Drug Abuse, 2001.

National Institute on Drug Abuse. (April 4, 1997). Genetic basis indicated for abuse of marijuana. Press release. http://www.os.dhhs.gov/news/press/1997pres/970404.html.

NBC News. (February 3, 1999). Coffee addiction may be genetic. Wysjg://18http. nbc739...s_archives/99-020307coffee. shml.

Nisbett, R.E. (1972). Hunger, obesity, and ventromedial hypothalamus. Psychological Review, vol. 79:433-453.

Parades, A., Hodd, W.R., Seymour, H. & Gollob, M. (1973). Loss of control in alcoholism: An investigation of the hypothesis, with experimental findings. Quarterly Journal of Studies on Alcohol, vol. 34:1141-1161.

Pargman, D. & Baker, M.C. (1980). Running high: Enkephalin indicted. Journal of Drug Issues, vol. 10:341-349

Partnership for a Drug-Free America. Partnership Attitude Tracking Study, 1999.

Peele, S. (1980). Addiction to an experience: A social-pharmacological theory of addiction. In D.J. Lettieri, M. Sayer, and H.W. Pearson, (Eds.). Theories of Drug Abuse. Research Monographs 30. Rockville, MD: National Institute on Drug Abuse.

Peele, S. (1983a). Is alcoholism different from other substance abuse? American Psychologist, vol. 38:963-964.

Peele, S., & Broadsky, A. (1975). Love and addiction. New York: Taplinger.

Pinderhughes, (1989). Understanding race, ethnicity, and power. Professional Counselor, October 1999.

Prochaska, J.O., & DiClemente, C.C. (1983). Stages and process of self-change of smoking: Toward an integrative model of change. Journal of Clinical Psychology, 5:390-395.

Robin, L.N., Davis, D.H. & Goodwin, D.W. (1978). Drug use by U.S. army enlisted men in Vietnam: A follow-up on their return home. American Journal of Epidemiology, vol. 99:235-249.

Roller, K. Pharmacotherapy commands increased attention in treatment of substance abuse, http://www.findarticle.com/cf_0/m3374/10_21/55090823/p1/article.jhtml, pp.1

Room, R., (1984). Alcohol control and public health. Annual Review of Public Health, vol. 5:293-317.

Rossing, M.A., (May 1998). Genetic Influence on Smoking: Candidate Genes. Environmental Health Perspective, vol. 106, No. 5.

Schaeffer, K.W., Paeson, O.A. & Yohman, Jr., (1984). Neurophysiological differences between male familial and non-familial alcoholics and nonalcoholics. Alcoholism Clinical Experience Research, vol. 8:347-351.

Schukit, M.A., & Rayses, V., (1979). Ethanol ingestion: Differences in blood acetaldehyde concentrations in relatives of alcoholics and control. Science, vol. 203:54-55.

Schukit, M.A., (1984b). Subjective responses to alcoholism in sons of alcoholics and control subjects. Archives of General Psychiatry, vol. 41:879-884.

Schukit, M.A., Goodwin, D.W., & Winokur, G., (1972). A study of alcoholism in half siblings. America Journal of Psychiatry, vol. 128:1132-1136.

Schultz, W.C. (1967). Joy. New York: Grove Press.

Science Daily Magazine, (April 26, 1999). Researchers find genetics connection to cigarette smoking.
http://www.sciencedaily.com/releases/1999/0199012608174.htm.

Shaffer, H.J. & Robbins, M. (1995). Psychotherapy for addictive behavior: A stage change approach to meaning making. In A.M. Washington (Eds.), psychotherapy and substance abuse: A practitioner's handbook. New York: Guilford Press.

Shaver, M. (October 8, 1999). Doctor sue insurer, claims sex addiction. Courier-Journal. http://www.courier-journal.com/loc.../1999/9910/08/991008addiction.htm.

Shkilnyk, A.M., (1984). A poison stronger than love: The destruction of an ojibawa community. New Haven, CT: Yale University.

Sichel, J., & Ellis, A. (1984). RET self-help form. New York: Institute for Rational-Emotive Therapy.

Sieber, M.F., & Angst, J. (1990). Alcohol, tobacco and cannabis: 12-year longitudinal association with antecedent social context and personality. Drug Alcohol Depend, 25:281-292.

Simkin, J.S. (1976). Gestalt therapy minilectures. Millbrae, CA: Celestial Arts.

Skidmore, J.E. (1993). A follow-up of therapist trained in the use of the solution-focused brief therapy model. Doctorial dissertation, University of South Dakota.

Sloboda, Z. Drug abuse in rural America: New solution to a growing problem. Counselor, December 2002.

Smith, D., (1981). The benzodiazepines and alcohol. Paper presented at Third World Congress of Biological Psychiatry, Stockholm.

Snyder, S.H., (1977). Opiate receptors and internal opiates. Scientific America, vol. 236 (No. 3):44-56.

Spillane, J., Did prohibition work? Reflections on the end of the first cocaine experience in the United States (pp.1), 1910-45. Journal of Drug Issues, Spring 1998.

Stunkard, A.J., et al. (1986). An adoption study of human obesity. New England Journal of Medicine, vol. 314:193-198.

Taleff, M.J. (1997). Solution-oriented and treatment: Similarities and differences. Alcohol Treatment Quarterly, 15 (1).

Tarter, R.E., Hegedus, A.M., Goldstein, G., Shelly, C., & Alterman, A.J., (1984). Adolescent sons of alcoholics: Neuropsychological and personal characteristics. Alcoholism Clinical Experience, vol. 8:216-222.

The Times of India, (January 27, 1999). Genes may be the culprit. http://www.indiatimes.com/news/more990127-01.html.

Tomkins, S. (1968). A modified model of smoking behavior. In E.F. Borgatta & R.R. Evans (Eds.). Smoking and health behavior (pp. 165-186). Chicago, IL: Aldine Publishing Company.

Wachuku, K., Ph.D. (2003). Anthology of monographs on addiction studies. Bloomington, IN: 1stBooks.

Waldorf, D., (1983). Natural recovery from opiate addiction: Some social-psychological processes of untreated recovery. Journal of Drug Issues, vol. 13:237-280.

Watzlawick, P. Weakland, J. & Fisch, R., (1974). Change: Principles of problem formation and problem resolution. New York: Norton.

What is solution-focused therapy? Harvard Mental Health Letter, April 1, 1997, vol. 13, Issue 10, pp. 8.

White, W. (1998). Slaying the dragon: The history of addiction treatment and recovery in America. Bloomington, IL: Chestnut Health System Publication.

Wicklund, R. & Brehm, J. (1998). Resistance to change: The cornerstone of cognitive dissonance theory. In E. Harmon-Jones and J.S. Mills, Cognitive dissonance theory: Revival with revisions and controversies. Washington, D.C.: America Psychological Association.

Yontef, G. (1969). Gestalt therapy: Its inheritance from gestalt psychology. Gestalt Theory, 4, 23-39.

Yontef, G. (1976). Gestalt: Clinical phenomenology. In V. Binder, A. Binder & R. Rimland (Eds.), Modern therapies (pp. 65-79). New York: Prentice Hall.

ABOUT THE AUTHOR

Dr. Kay Wachuku received his bachelor's degree in Mass Communication from Hampton University, Hampton, Virginia, in 1983. In 1985 he received his master's degree in Education from Southern University, Baton Rouge, Louisiana. He has been an educator for over sixteen years, serving as professor of Journalism for three years and subsequently teaching as adjunct instructor. Dr. Wachuku received a doctorate degree in Addictive Disorders from the College for Advanced Studies in Addictive Disorders, Breining Institute, Orangevale, California. While teaching at Juvenile Court Schools in San Bernardino, California, in 1987 he began making a connection between substance abuse and juvenile hall incarceration. Subsequently, he began investigating the role of substance abuse and juvenile/youth dysfunction. In 1992, he launched the first multi-family unit substance abuse aftercare treatment program in San Bernardino County. The concept was to house successful graduates from local substance abuse treatment programs in four separate apartment complexes. Each complex was equipped with a twelve-step meeting hall. Residents received on-going relapse prevention education and counseling. All residents in the apartments were drug and alcohol free. The program was an instant success. About 85 percent of the 450 residents remained sober and had gainful employment past one year after admission into the program. In 1995, NBC primetime news dubbed the program "Sober Living at its Best." Dr. Wachuku directed the youth Substance abuse treatment program (TEAP) for the Inland Empire Job Corps in San Bernardino, California for six years. Dr. Wachuku pioneered more innovation in the Inland Empire Job Corps substance abuse program than his predecessors and colleagues among the 118 Job Corps centers nation wide. In April 2002, the Department of Labor (funding source for the Job Corps Program) reviewers rated the Inland Empire Job Corps substance abuse program best in the nation. He was a favored trainer for the Job Corps National Health and Wellness Conferences and the National TEAP bi-annual Conference. Dr. Wachuku is the author of *TEAP Relapse Prevention Workbook and Anthology of Monographs on Addiction Studies*. He has appeared in many local television programs and more recently he appeared on the TBN "Joy in our Town" program discussing issues in substance abuse. He is a drug-free community activist, a mentor and a married father of four children.